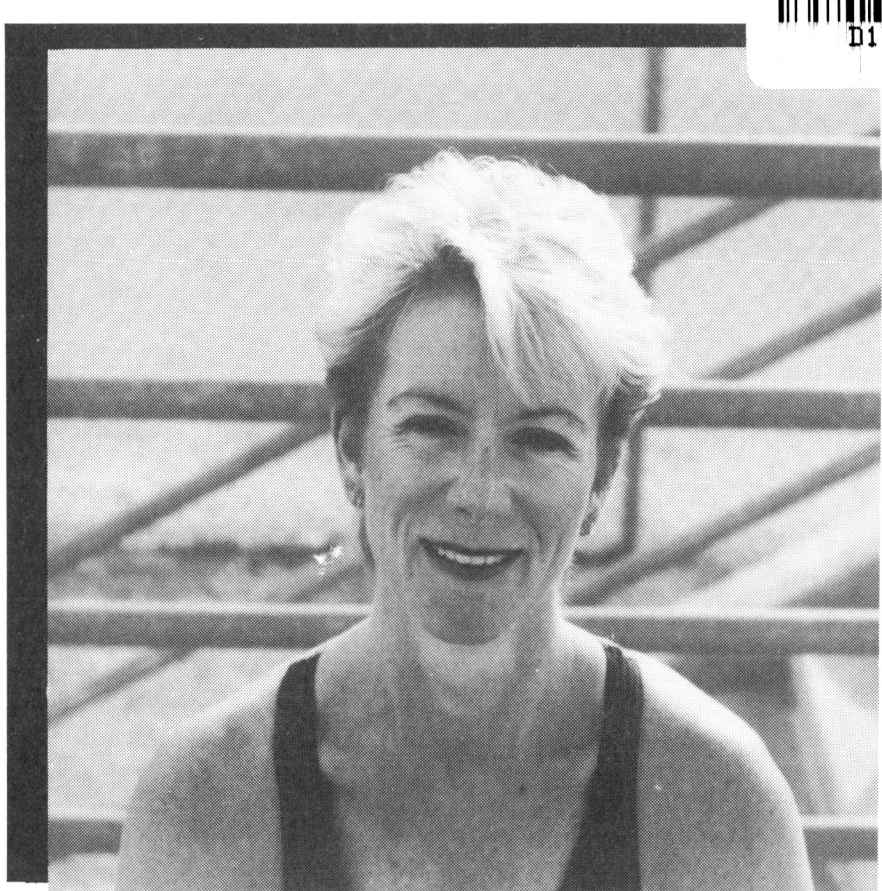

KATE MONTGOMERY

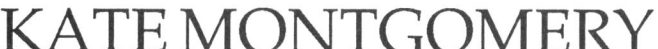

Certified Sports Massage Therapist
Certified Respiratory Therapist

SPORTS TOUCH

P. O. Box 229002 – 155
San Diego, CA 92122

SPORTS TOUCH ®

THE ATHLETIC RITUAL

Published by
SPORTS TOUCH ®
P.O. Box 229002-155
San Diego, CA 92122

Library of Congress Cataloging in Publication Data

Montgomery, Kate, 1951 –
    Sports touch : the athletic ritual / Kate Montgomery. —
    p. cm.
    Includes bibliographical references and index.
    ISBN 1-878069-00-4

    1. Physical education and training.   2. Sports medicine.
    3. Physical fitness.   I. Title.
GV711.5   796

                                              QBI91-314

"SPORTS TOUCH®" and its Flamingo Logo are registered
with the U.S. Patent and Trademark Office.

First Printing March, 1990 • Second Printing June, 1991

THE SECRET WEAPON OF THE 90'S

THE ATHLETIC RITUAL is the *SECRET WEAPON* which enables you to **recover with record-breaking speed — and the results are** *immediate!*

This system is a **MUST** for any athlete who seeks to attain peak performance. And for those who compete in either amateur or professional events, these rituals provide the critical edge, *which makes the difference between winning and losing.*

At the 1989 Ironman Triathlon in Kona, Hawaii, Montgomery's athletes recovered in an unheard of 24 – 72 hours!

"The next day I felt fine — absolutely fantastic — already thinking about next year! Gauging by what I feel was an unbelievable recovery, I would recommend these techniques to anyone."

Joe Kilmer
1989 Ironman, Kona

"My swim time is usually 1:10 to 1:20. To my surprise, I did it in one hour flat and I felt great"

John Carey
1989 Ironman, Kona

"After exhausting all avenues of conventional treatment... I turned to Kate and her methods... which I used in the Olympic Games in Seoul. Not only did we win the Gold Medal, but my energy level didn't wane during the entire 21 days.

"You have nothing to lose but a few minutes a day, and you have oh, so much to gain!"

Bob Ctvrtlik
1988 USA Volleyball Team
Gold Medal Winner
Seoul Olympic Games

Although I developed this book especially for athletes, *it will benefit everyone,* for we are all athletes at some level. From the homemaker who bends, stoops, and lifts all day, to the high-stress executive, to children and seniors, we all engage in some sort of physical activity, and we all must cope with various forms of stress. Anyone can apply these techniques and create a better functioning and more energized body and mind.

Kate Montgomery
Author & Sports Massage Therapist

Dedicated to...

This book is dedicated to Bess James. Her spirit, dedication to life, always climbing the highest peak, courage and never-give-up attitude have inspired my life. The love, caring and encouragement she has given me are more than I can express. She is one of a kind! I love you, Bess.

Always your friend and daughter —

Kate

ACKNOWLEDGEMENTS

From the inception of this book, I have had a lot of love, support, and encouragement from some wonderful people. If it hadn't been for these friends believing in me and giving of themselves so generously, I don't know how I would have gotten through.

Thank you Jim Powry, who created the format for this book along with his valuable time, and to Bob Liebman who took over for Jim and brought me further toward my goal. Judy Smith and her wonderful illustrations for the acupressure portion of the book plus all her generous time she has given to this project. To Kathy Upton and Michael Delgado for all their wonderful support and encouragement. To Greg Creswell who as a "hobby," provided most of the book's wonderful illustrations and graphics, thank you for sharing your wonderful talent.

Next to all my contributors who over the last five years enriched my knowledge about healing — your contribution was priceless.

To the Institute of Psycho-Structural Balancing, who taught me a more healthful way to live.

Thank you Deborah Walker, D.C., for your love and support and for introducing me to the principles of applied kinesiology, and to Craig Dillman, D.C. who helped me refine my Rituals and was always there when I needed him. A special thanks to Rick Gold, Acupuncturist, who taught me how to use pressure points to release blocked energy and to make my clients whole and healthy again. For introducing me to a way of assessing the body as a whole not as a part.

Thank you to Jeri Nielson, who pounded her fingers to the bone getting this manuscript typed and ready to go.

Many, many thanks to Beverly Trainer, who spent long hours editing this material — I couldn't have done it without you!

To David Hemingway, who posed for all the pictures. Whenever I needed him, he was there. Thank you for believing in my system and being the first to try it. To Brad Yeater, my photographer — for all your time and patience. Thank you.

To Tony Allen-Cooksey, my friend and trainer who taught me how to "listen" to an athlete. For helping me to put the chapter on stretching together —thank you.

ACKNOWLEDGEMENTS

To all the Athletes who — without hesitation — were willing to try my system and prove its validity with fantastic results — a very special thank you and to all my clients who let me practice on them to set my techniques"just right", thank you from the bottom of my heart.

Finally, all my friends who were always there for me when I needed encouragement,, — you were terrific!

A very special thank you to my daughter Carissa, for being so understanding and patient during these last two years. I love you.

This book has truly been a labor of love, for my heart and soul are in this "Ritual." I truly believe in its power to change lives, and it thrills me when I see athletes making break throughs they never believed were possible.

I hope that you too, will try the Ritual, for it's the only way you can personally experience its results.

To each one of you who is willing to take responsibility for your life and increase your energy, performance and overall health and happiness — this book is for you!

THE ATHLETIC RITUAL
TOPICS

THE ATHLETIC RITUAL
TOPICS

THE SPORTS TOUCH RITUAL
INTRODUCTION

Ritual -- Webster's Dictionary defines the term as "any formed and customarily repeated act or series of acts." [1]

Rituals are not an exotic practice, but rather something we all do — unconsciously — every day. A habit as simple as brushing your teeth after each meal is a form of ritual, and one which is necessary for good dental health.

Other rituals are psychological and their repetition serves to either relax or energize us as we prepare for challenging events. For example, have you ever watched a ball player as he steps up to the plate? He may make the sign of the cross or say a quick prayer to himself before he takes his stance. While his prayer may or may not be answered, the familiarity of the "ritual" helps provide him with a comfort zone.

We all have our own particular rituals whether we are conscious of them or not, so I've created a few specific ones you can add for maintaining and improving your health.

This book is about creating, through a sequence of steps, your own ritual to energize and strengthen your body while it enhances your immune system.

One of the hidden values of these rituals is the improvement of mind/body coordination. As you do them on a regular basis, you'll begin to feel stronger and notice a positive change in your hand – eye coordination. You also should detect an improvement in your mental acuity.

A complex condition known as dyslexia involves neurological disorganization. Most people associate dyslexia with learning disabilities, but it also affects muscular coordination. Severe dyslexic problems should be handled by a qualified professional, but simple muscular uncoordination could possibly be corrected by doing these techniques every day.

Although I developed this book especially for athletes, it will benefit everyone, for we are all athletes at some level. From the homemaker who bends, stoops, and lifts all day, to the high-stress executive, to children and seniors, we all engage in some sort of physical activity, and we all must cope with various forms of stress. Anyone can apply these techniques and create a better functioning and more energized body and mind.

It is important to begin every ritual with **Diaphragm Breathing** and **Release** (*if necessary*), **Sacral Rock**, and **Respiratory Spinal Extension**. After that you may proceed to the other steps in the order given. It is particularly important to keep these steps in sequence when competing in an athletic event, to achieve your highest levels of endurance and stamina.

[1.] **Webster's New World Dictionary, Second College Edition.**

DYNAMICS OF BREATHING

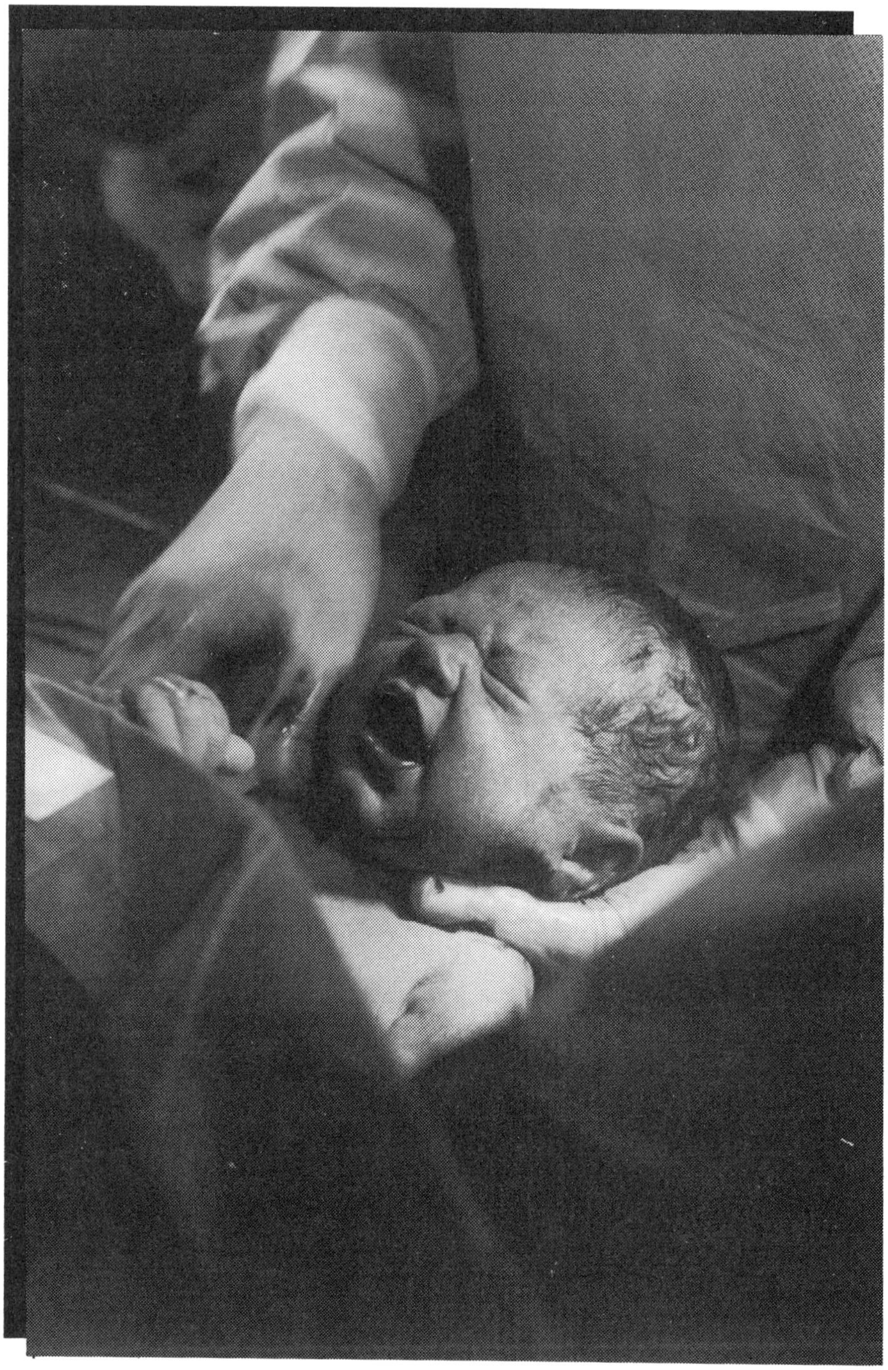

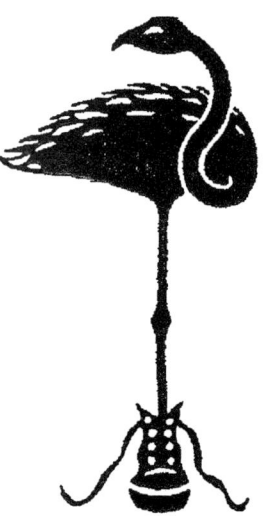

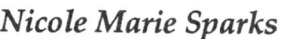

Nicole Marie Sparks

OUR FIRST BREATH

Meet Nicole Marie Sparks. This photograph shows her taking her very first breath! Only moments old, Nicole's body knows only one way to breathe — using the muscle specifically designed to assist her breathing: The Diaphragm. This muscle has been the most over-looked muscle in the body, and the most difficult to evaluate and treat.

Other than the heart, THE DIAPHRAGM IS THE BODY'S MOST IMPORTANT AND PRIMARY MUSCLE.

There are many symptomatic problems which result from a non-functioning diaphragm muscle. These include shortness of breath after minimal exercise, chronic fatigue, nausea following running, a stitch or cramp in your side during exercise, and structural imbalance of the spine which leads to a possible decrease of nerve reflex activity in the diaphragm muscle.

One or more of these symptoms would indicate a need for diaphragm testing. By reestablishing proper diaphragm activity, you can improve breathing capacity, increase oxygenation to the muscles, nerves and organs, enhance mental and physical relaxation, and reestablish a connection to the autonomic nervous system.

After that, you may proceed to other steps in the order given. Eventually, you will be able to create your own SPORTS TOUCH RITUAL, tailored specifically to your own needs, and this program will enable you to achieve your highest levels of endurance and stamina.

BREATHING FOR BETTER HEALTH & ENERGY

Breathing...

It sounds easy — something so natural and automatic that we take it for granted. Yet, the importance of breathing is understated; our very existence depends on it. But did you know that you can improve each breath you take? All you need is one simple alteration: simply use your diaphragm muscle.

But perhaps you're asking, "Why **should** I change the way I breathe?" The reason involves efficiency. You can increase your lung volume by approximately 200 cc's, according to your body size and weight. I've determined this figure by using a simple spirometer, which measures the amount of air inhaled. First, I measure the inspired volume when my client uses only his chest muscles; then I teach him to breathe using the diaphragm along with the other respiratory muscles. There is usually an approximate increase of 200 cc's of inspired volume, simply by changing the method of breathing.

What this means to you is that you are now able to increase the amount of oxygen going to your muscles and other body tissues more efficiently. The body's normal levels of pH, carbon dioxide, and oxygen are affected by changes in our breathing pattern. Especially too shallow breathing, which is called hyperventilation. If we "shallow breathe" too long or even over a period of years, many changes can occur. The carbon dioxide in the blood is reduced. It is a waste by-product of respiration and is responsible for maintaining the pH balance of our blood. Breathing too fast, we "blow off" this carbon dioxide before it can do its job. Hyperventilation causes the blood vessels to constrict, preventing sufficient oxygen from reaching the muscles — oxygen which is needed to handle the increased demands of exercise. This phenomenon will lead to a feeling of "burning" in your legs. (Example: You have been out running and 30 minutes into it, your legs start to burn and get heavy; you start to slow down and become increasingly tired.)

A build-up of the waste by-product, lactic acid, will also cause a decrease in the flow of calcium into the tissues, caused by the change in the blood's pH level. Because calcium is a natural muscle relaxer, deficiency will produce hypersensitive muscles. You may even feel nervous, shaky, and anxious; your hands and feet may become tingly and even cold. Feelings of confusion (lack of oxygen to the brain), disorientation, and impaired memory and emotional instability may result.

BREATHING FOR BETTER HEALTH & ENERGY

Unfortunately, most people breathe from their chest, and that is the most inefficient way to take in oxygen. Chest breathing requires more effort to accomplish the ventilation/perfusion (air to blood mix), resulting in an increased respiratory rate, and increased stress on the heart. Chest breathing also encourages what is called the Flight/Fight Syndrome, a result of prolonged hyperventilation.

Increased tension, anxiety, restlessness, and shallow breathing are all caused by stress. We don't always realize or notice the change in our pattern of breathing during stressful situations. Replacing the breathing pattern with diaphragmatic breathing creates a deeper sense of relaxation and increases clarity of mind. The body becomes less tense as the muscles relax.

And as you might imagine, there is a change in athletic performance too. Decreased agility, alertness, coordination, early fatigue, decreased strength, stamina and endurance can all be reversed by Diaphragmatic Breathing.

The benefits of Diaphragmatic Breathing are well worth the small effort required. Each diaphragmatic breath you take makes you feel calmer, your memory is sharper (the better to make those last minute adjustments in the long jump), and you will have more energy, better coordination, better stamina and endurance to complete your tasks at hand. There are other internal benefits to Diaphragmatic Breathing that most of us are not aware of.

"The pericardium, the sac surrounding the heart, is attached to the diaphragm. As you breathe deeply, the diaphragm descends, stretching the heart downward toward the abdomen. When the lungs become filled, the heart receives a gentle massage. As the diaphragm relaxes, it also massages the liver and pancreas, and helps to improve functions of the spleen, stomach and small intestine."[1] This gentle massage, that only you can give yourself, aids in better digestion, elimination, heart function, augmenting respiration and blood and lymphatic circulation to aid in eliminating toxic substances, which make your body feel sluggish and uncomfortable. This is an instance when you can be your own therapist — easy! Wow! What a wonderful gift you have given yourself! And all because you learned how to diaphragmatically breathe, the way nature intended.

[1]**Science of Breathe**, 1979, The Himalayan International Institute of Yoga, Science and Philosophy, Honesdale, Pennsylvania.

THE DYNAMICS OF BREATHING
MUSCULATURE INVOLVED

The primary muscle involving inspiration is the diaphragm. It is a parachute-like sheet of muscle, which is innervated by the phrenic nerve (vagus nerve) to produce stimulation and movement along the lower rib cage. It resembles a parachute because when it's filled with air, it billows, and it flattens again as it deflates. As you inhale, the diaphragm contracts, and descends downward and outward decreasing the size of the abdominal cavity. The rib cage then lifts and moves outward, increasing the size of the chest/thoracic cavity. Other muscles involved in inspiration are the intercostals, which lie between the ribs, connecting them, and slope both downward and forward. When you inhale, the intercostals also contract, pulling the ribs upward and forward.

Accessary muscles are the scalene or neck muscles. They help to lift the first two ribs and the sternum. In shallow, restful breathing, they produce very little movement. But during exercise, these are the muscles which cause the nostrils to flare and the neck muscles to contract and work vigorously.

When you breathe normally, expiration is a passive movement. The chest wall and lung are elastic and recoil voluntarily after inspiration. The most important muscles here are the abdominals. When they contract, the diaphragm is pushed upward, decreasing the size of the chest cavity as the abdominal cavity enlarges.

Accessory muscles of expiration are called internal intercostals. In exercise they assist in active expiration by forcibly pulling the ribs downward and inward. This action decreases the volume in the chest cavity.

DYNAMICS OF BREATHING

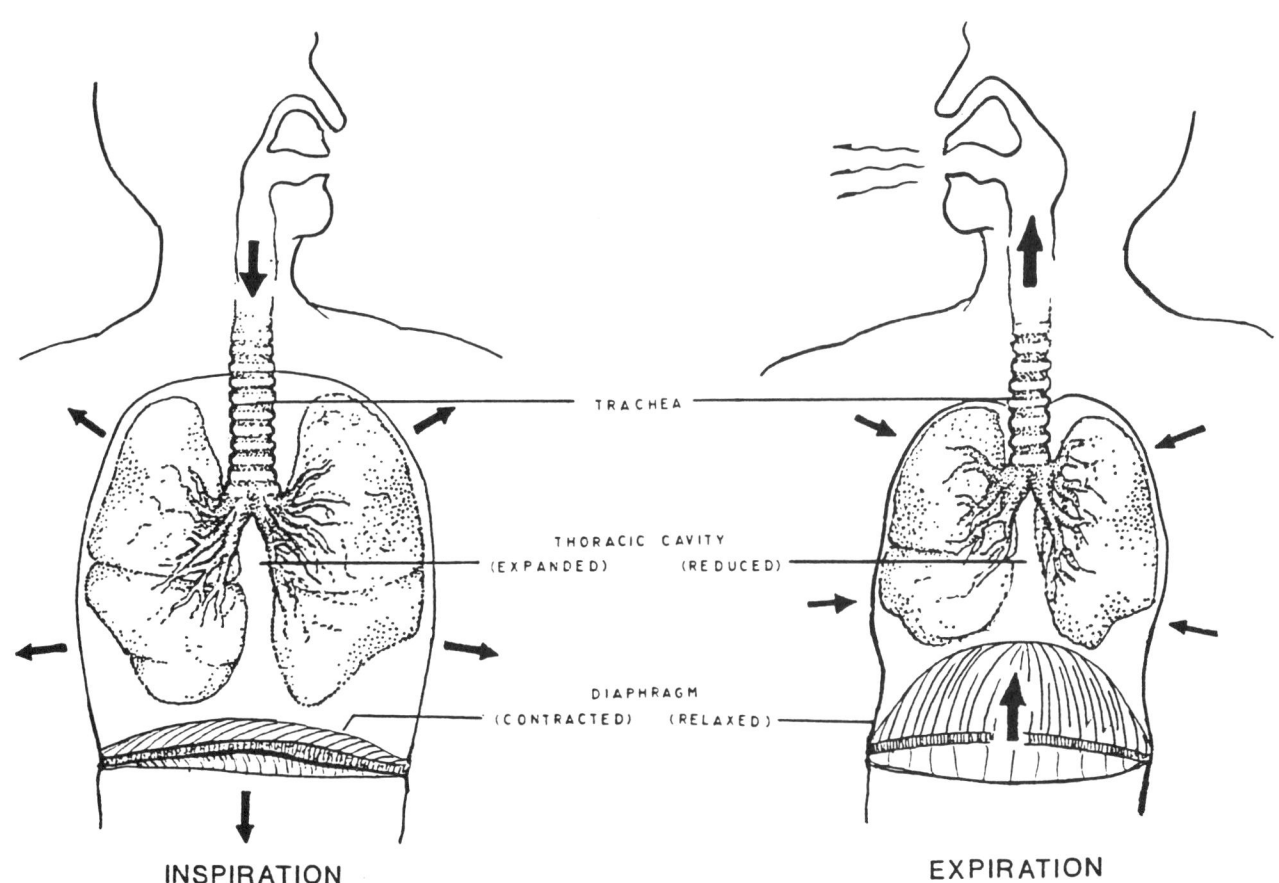

TRACHEA

THORACIC CAVITY
(EXPANDED)   (REDUCED)

DIAPHRAGM
(CONTRACTED)   (RELAXED)

INSPIRATION   EXPIRATION

Illustration by Greg Creswell

THE DYNAMICS OF BREATHING
MUSCULATURE INVOLVED

Our lungs are quite a wonder — they supply our body with enough oxygen, carbon dioxide and other gases to regulate our entire metabolism. Treated with respect and care, they will last a life time. And by learning how to fully utilize the efficiency of our lungs, as nature intended, we can create a better physical and mental well-being.

When shallow breathing (hyperventilation) occurs over long periods of time, lack of oxygen occurs, it can produce pre-mature aging of our brain through loss of brain cells which contribute to memory loss and senility.

When we are born, diaphragmatic breathing is automatic. But as we adopt improper breathing habits, all these muscles become weak with disuse, and atrophy sets in.

Fortunately, it can be reversed. Through diaphragmatic breathing, you can restrengthen and regenerate your muscles so that they can function as naturally and efficiently as the day you were born.

DIAPHRAGMATIC BREATHING:
WHAT YOU ARE FEELING

What you are feeling when trying to learn Diaphragmatic Breathing:

Learning to do Diaphragmatic Breathing isn't as easy as it appears. When you first start to change your breathing pattern, you may feel awkward and frustrated. Don't give up. You are reprogramming your brain (your computer) to breathe differently. As you move the air upward, starting from the abdominal area, your abdomen protrudes outward. As the air rises, you may feel a "catch" in which the air doesn't go where you want it to. A "catch" as I call it is the areas in the lungs that haven't been ventilated or opened up fully. As you take that first deep breath, you may feel like you are on a "roller coaster," traveling first to the chest, then back down to the stomach, and then back up again. Or feeling only one side of the lung open up better than the other. Your lungs are made up of tiny tubes, called bronchioles, and at the end of these tubes are tiny air sacs called alveoli. These sacs are like little balloons, waiting there to be inflated with oxygen. These sacs help with the distribution of oxygen into our blood that moves it into our muscles, organs and brain. When this system doesn't work as efficiently as it could, it leaves us feeling fatigued, short of breath during exercise, run down and just not enough energy to propel us through our day.

Those "catches" I spoke of earlier will gradually disappear as you practice Diaphragmatic Breathing. A fluid, even flowing feeling of air will move upward, spreading throughout your lungs without hesitation. The more you focus on how you breathe, the more aware you will become of developing a more efficient breathing system.

DIAPHRAGMATIC BREATHING
HOW TO DIAPHRAGMATICALLY BREATHE

Before you begin, seek out a quiet place to lie down. When you are comfortable and relaxed, place your hands on your upper abdomen, just below the rib cage, and focus on this area.

I.   As you inhale, push your abdomen outward, and feel the air rise upward to your chest, then rise further up to your shoulder area. Each breath should be fluid and relaxed.

II. Exhale passively, then begin again. Of course, like any exercise, this may feel awkward at first, but with practice and concentration, you can retrain yourself to breathe only diaphragmatically — the way nature intended. (Pg. 11)

INSPIRATION / EXPIRATION DIAGRAM

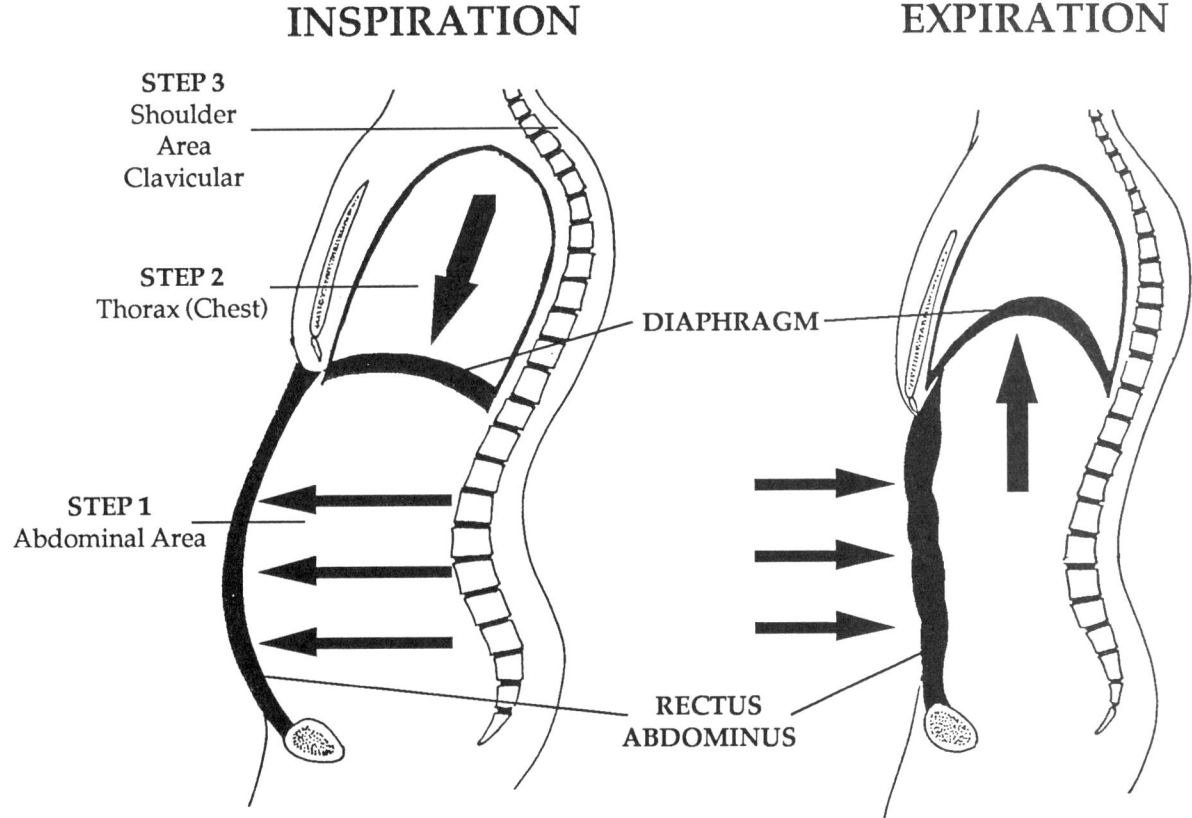

INSPIRATION   **EXPIRATION**

STEP 3
Shoulder
Area
Clavicular

STEP 2
Thorax (Chest)

DIAPHRAGM

STEP 1
Abdominal Area

RECTUS
ABDOMINUS

Illustration by Greg Creswell

THE ATHLETE

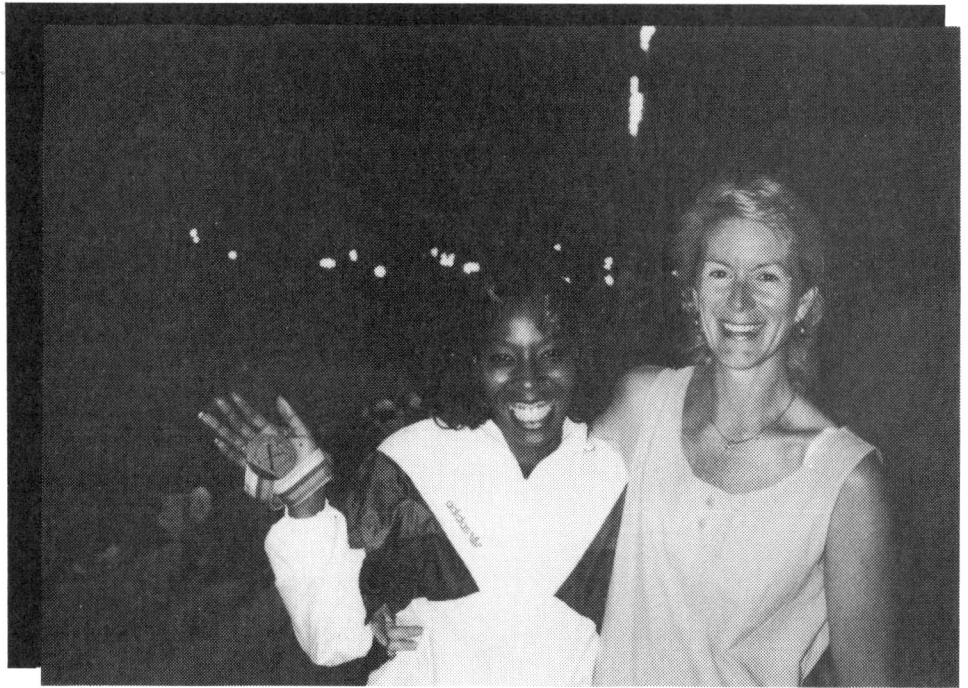

LaTanya Sheffield and myself

1987 Pan American Games
LaTanya was the Bronze Medal Winner
in the 400 meter hurdles.

THE ATHLETE

This method of **diaphragmatic release** is perfectly tailored for the athlete who needs to gain maximum strength, stamina, and endurance. The best thing about this technique is that you can do it yourself.

Have you ever experienced unpleasant symptoms during or after an event? **Nausea following a competition and cramps in the side which force you to slow down**. These are **completely eliminated** by Diaphagmatic Breathing and **Release**.

To stress the importance of this method, I'd like to tell you about a female 400-meter hurdler with whom I've worked. In 1987, at the Mobil Track and Field Championships in San Jose, I met La Tanya Sheffield, who just happened to be from San Diego, California. She told me that she had a history of becoming nauseated after every race, and when I muscle-tested her, I found that every major muscle was noticeably weak. I noticed also that La Tanya did not diaphragmatically breathe. Later that evening I explained diaphragmatic breathing and its importance to her running. I then taught her how to breathe properly, released her diaphragm, balanced all the major muscles in her body, especially those pertaining to her event, and finished the evening with a light massage.

Up to this time she had been extremely fatigued and had not been sleeping well. But once her body was balanced, La Tanya became a new person.

The finals of the 400-meter hurdles was the next day, and La Tanya was flying, breaking her personal records for speed. At the end of the race, she wasn't even tired, and most important, she wasn't nauseated. La Tanya went on to win the gold at the Olympic Festival in North Carolina that year, took the bronze at the Pan American Games in Indianapolis, and in 1988 made the USA Olympic Team for Seoul, South Korea.

By simply learning to breathe correctly and reactivating the **Diaphragm Muscle**, a whole new breath of fresh air and energy can be yours, and like La Tanya, you too may find yourself achieving new goals.

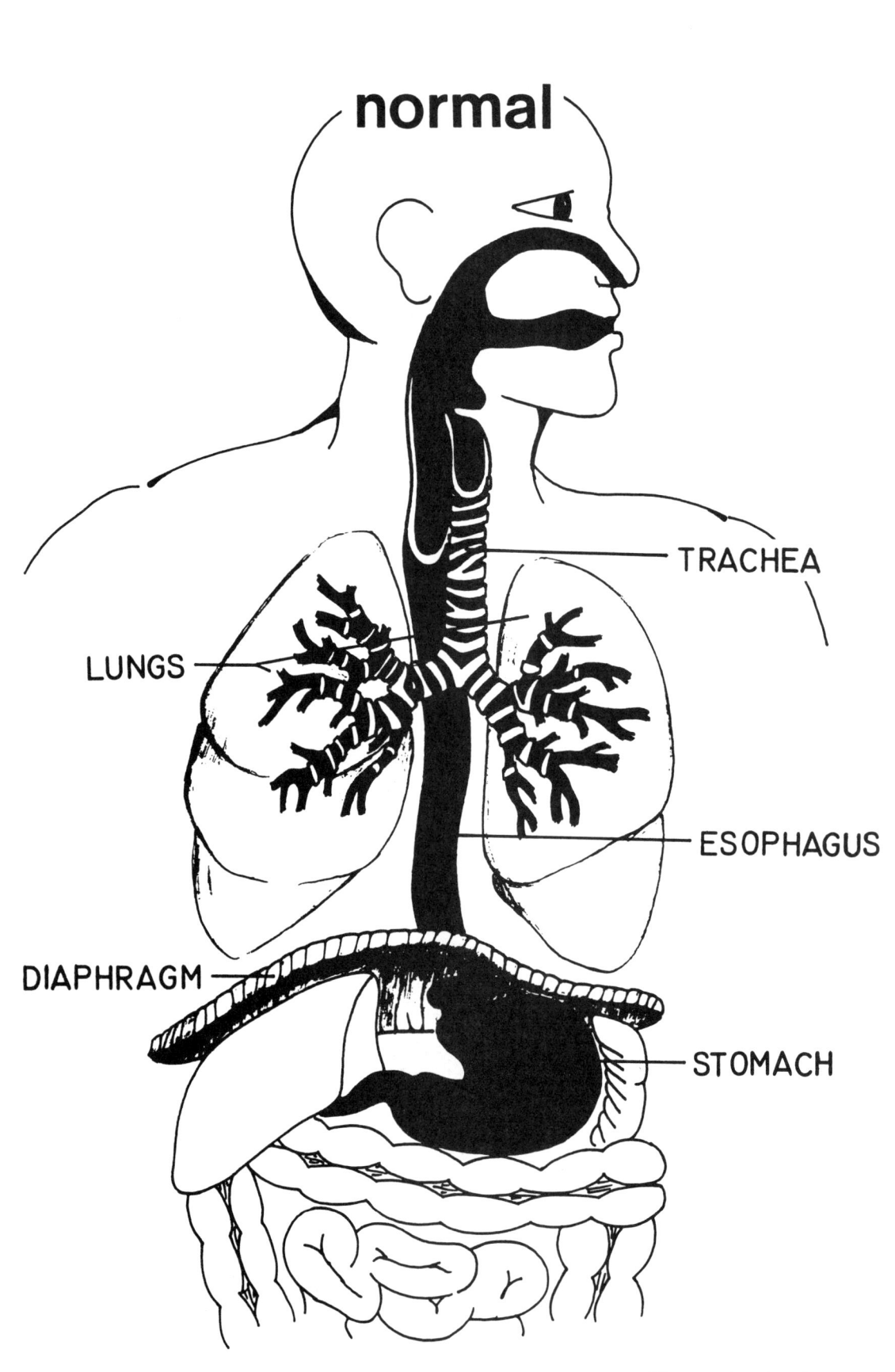

normal

TRACHEA

LUNGS

ESOPHAGUS

DIAPHRAGM

STOMACH

Illustration by Greg Creswell

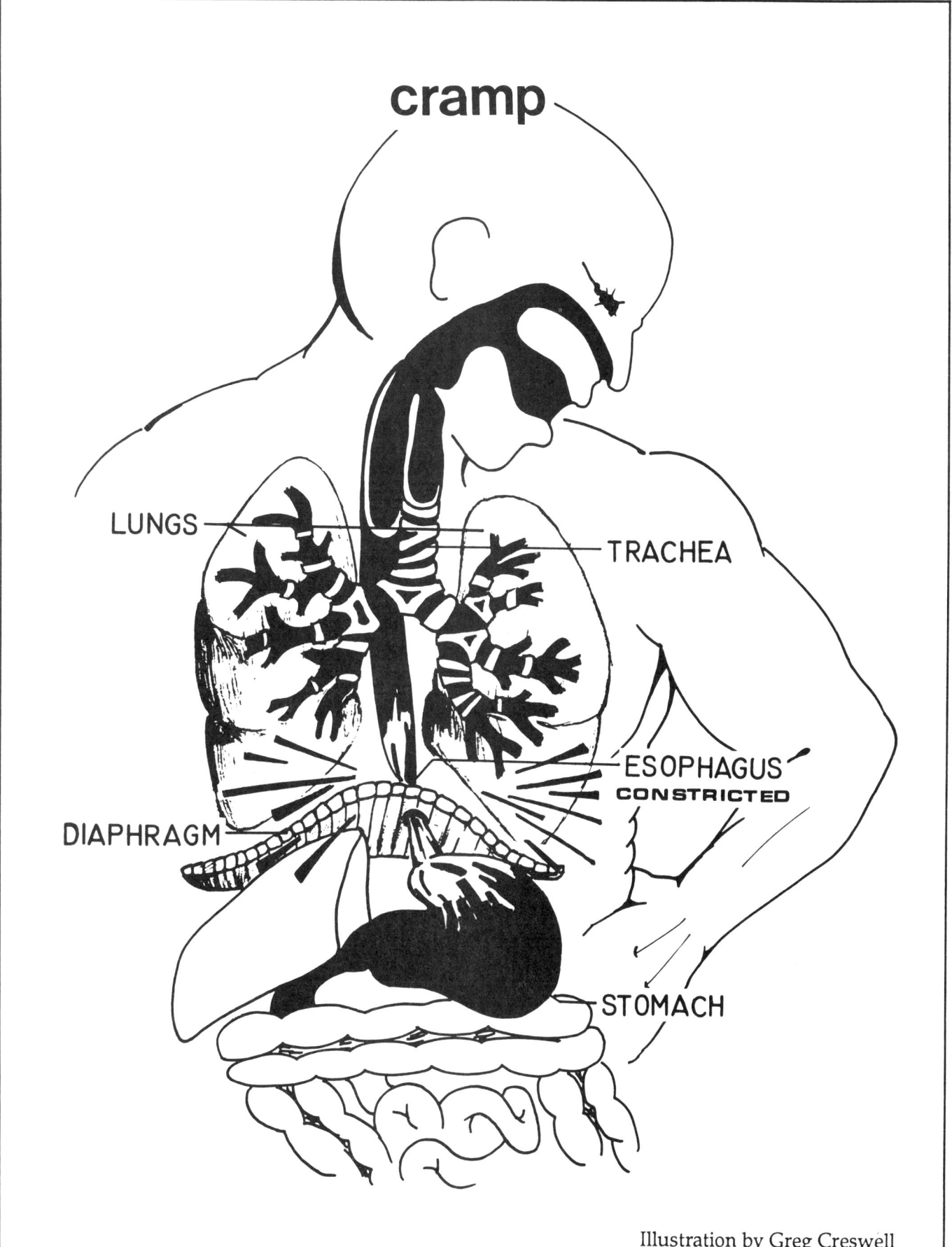

cramp

LUNGS

TRACHEA

ESOPHAGUS
CONSTRICTED

DIAPHRAGM

STOMACH

Illustration by Greg Creswell

THE ATHLETE

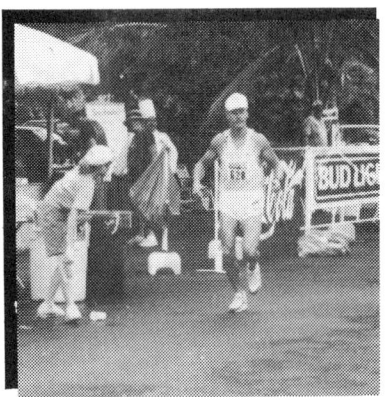

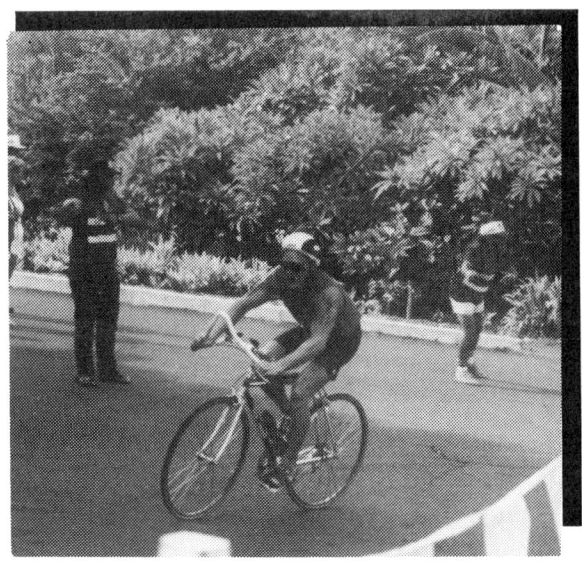

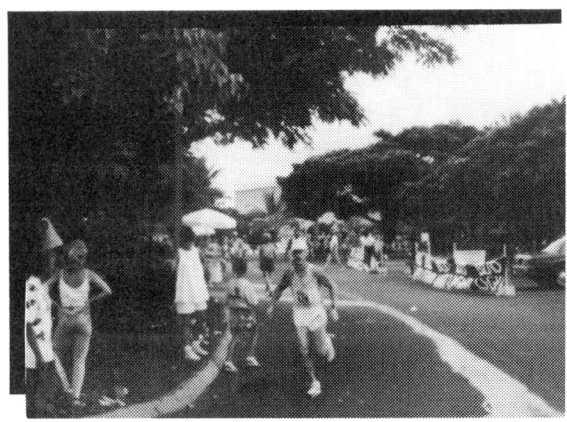

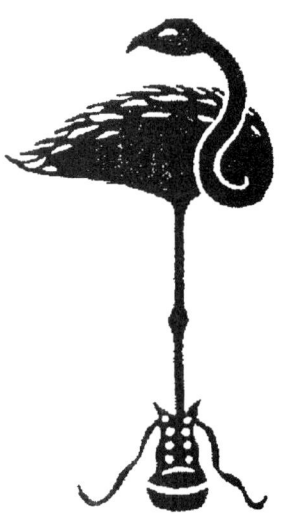

Joe Kilmer
Ironman
Oct. 14, 1989
Kona, Hawaii

APPLIED KINESIOLOGY – MUSCLE TESTING

"Applied Kinesiology concerns itself with balancing the structural, chemical, and psychological aspects of the individual.

"Through applied kinesiology techniques, we are able to access how the body's muscles and organs are functionally performing — both good and bad. It is particularly useful for sports related injuries because it can help find a muscle imbalance, weakness, or excessive tightness and balance the problem.

"Because the muscles and organs have an intimate connection, improving one assists the well being of the other in a reciprocal fashion."

Craig Dillman
Chiropractor
San Diego, CA

MUSCLE TESTING

The science of applied kinesiology was developed by Dr. George Goodheart, D.C., in the early 1960's. His theories generated a whole new way of working muscles that were tight or in spasm. There were indications that agonist muscles (muscles opposite one another) either showed weakness or excess strength in relationship to the other, which can cause eventual pain and can pull the spine out of alignment, creating tension throughout the body.

The development of muscle testing, or what I call a "bio-feedback" system between the mind and the body, is a simple way of testing a muscle for both strength and efficiency. By using special techniques, you can correct any imbalance.

When you test a muscle and it "goes weak," it is functioning at less than 100% capacity. There is a "short circuit" in the energy of the muscle which needs to be corrected so it can work at its maximum level. The nerves that innervate the muscles give the muscle its actual strength and power that it can produce. So it is really the nervous system we are dealing with. Applied kinesiology is directed at correcting structural imbalance caused by poorly functioning muscles.

Research is on going in kinesiology at the International College of Applied Kinesiology, "an organization of physicians whose main purpose is to improve and expand the scientific use of Applied Kinesiology in determining the cause of health problems."[2]

---

[2] **Applied Kinesiology — Synopsis**, *David S. Walther*, Systems, D.C., Pueblo, Colorado.

MUSCLE TESTING

WHY SHOULD YOU USE MUSCLE TESTING?

Muscle testing is a unique and immediate method of assessing what is "out-of-balance" in your body. For example: if you are training day after day without rest, your muscles will start to feel heavy and sluggish as they become over-worked. When this happens, you start to make slight muscular adjustments, eventually leading to a structural change down the road. One side of your body may begin to compensate by working harder than the other, thus creating a "lop-sided" effect. When muscles tighten, tendonitis can eventually develop, causing added stress and strain in the relationship of muscle to bone.

As the body shifts, compensation/misalignment takes place. When an athlete puts in hours and hours of training, stressing his legs and back and not getting enough rest without massage therapy to encourage muscular recovery, the body will eventually wear down and become vulnerable to injury.

Muscle testing is a tool, and when used on a regular basis along with other modes of therapy can prevent both injury and the deterioration.

HOW TO MUSCLE TEST

The athlete faces the therapist with one arm out-stretched at his or her side. The therapist, using two fingers, asks the athlete to hold his arm stiff, elbow locked. Then the therapist asks the athlete to inhale, and, as he exhales, the therapist applies pressure at the wrist in a downward motion. The athlete must not "strong-arm" the hold, but simply allow the arm to fall when he can no longer easily hold the position. We are taught to always be strong and so when asked to hold a position, we will "strain" to keep from being weak. If you have to strain, you are "strong-arming" the hold. Any muscle in the body can be used as an indicator muscle to achieve a response.

What the therapist is looking for is a "locked-in" muscle. A "locked-in" muscle is a muscle that is being tested and is applied the slightest pressure in a particular position and doesn't waiver. It holds strong. (Example: As in a door that is locked and does not move the slightest.) If the muscle is not locked-in, a "turned-off response" is indicated. What you will feel in a "turned-off response" is a feeling of weakness and a sense of not being able to hold the muscle taut without straining. (Pg. 21)

MUSCLE TESTING
FOR A HYPERTONIC DIAPHRAM

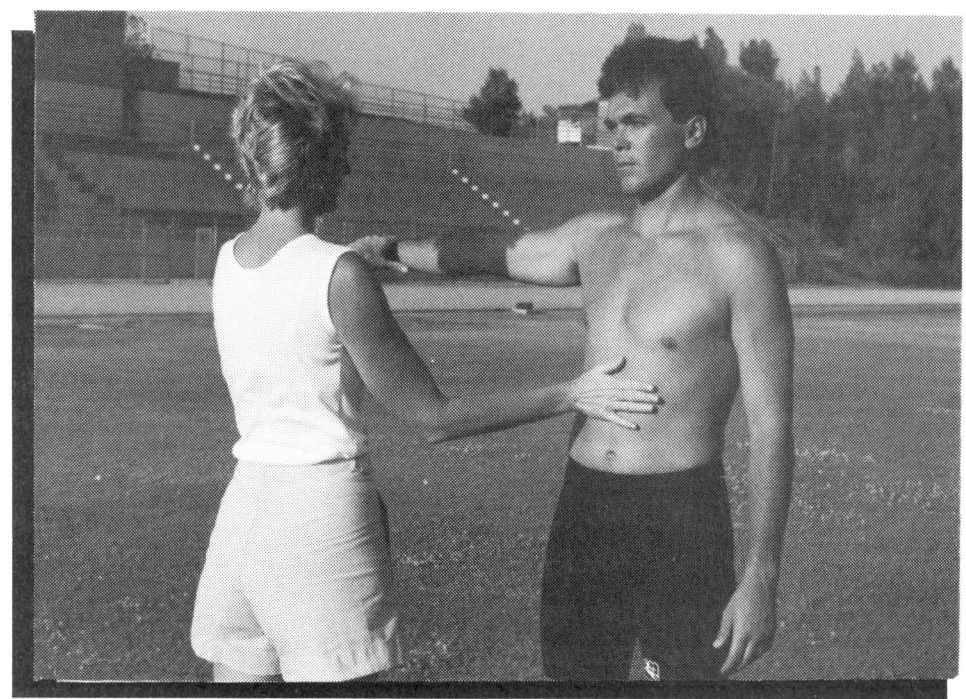

Figure A

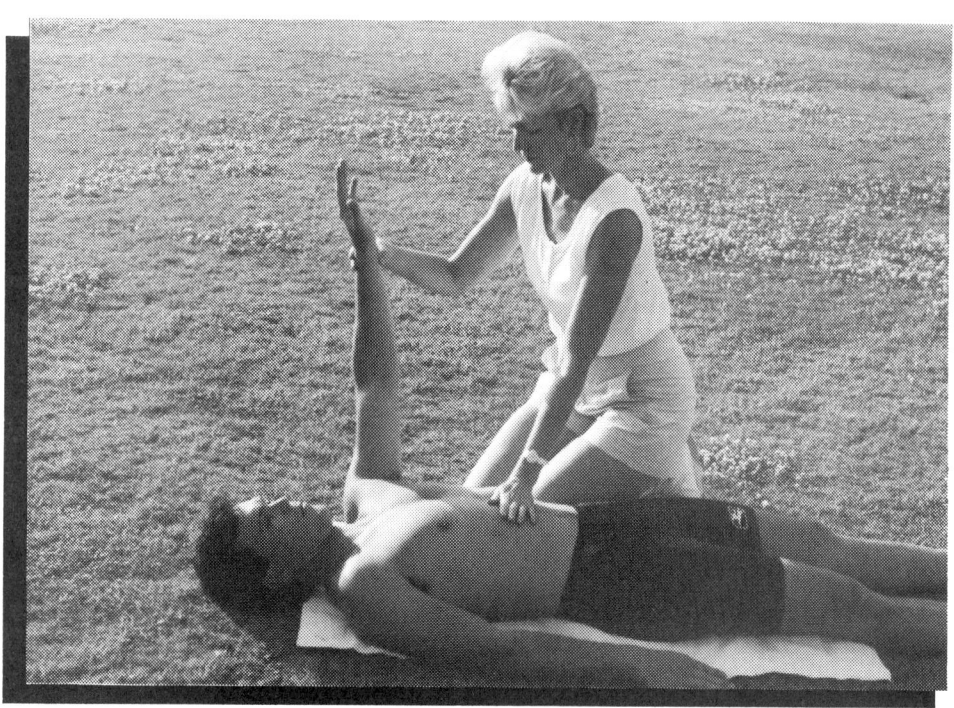

DIAPHRAGM RELEASE METHOD

The **diaphragm muscle**, due to its inactive state, is **hypertonic**. A hypertonic diaphragm is a muscle that has been in a contracted state due to non-use. Even though you diaphragmatically breathe, not all of the muscle fibers will release and become active again. You can release these muscle fibers by performing the **Diaphragm Release Method** (pictured on pg. 23).

HOW TO RELEASE THE DIAPHRAGM:

The athlete may either stand or lie down for this maneuver.

1. Standing or lying down, the athlete **inhales** diaphragmatically, all the way to the top of the shoulders, then

2. Holds his breath, and

3. Pushes his abdominal muscles outward and holds them taut ...

4. Then takes his hands and places his fingertips at the apex of the rib cage. (The apex is one-hands width moving laterally from the sternum — breastbone.) Still holding his breath, he pushes **gently** in and down along the rib cage, moving toward his side. This maneuver takes only seconds to do. Now **exhale**.

This enables you to avoid the ZIPHOID PROCESS located at the end of the sternum, which sometimes curves inward. **I repeat, you must push the abdominals outward and hold them taut. FAILURE TO DO THIS COULD PUNCTURE A LUNG OR SPLEEN.**

Have a friend muscle test you as described on pg. 20. **Inhale**, hold your breath, push abdominal muscle out and hold taut. At the same time, hold your arm out to your side, and have your friend's hand touch your abdomen while his other hand (two fingers) is at your wrist, **gently** pushing down on your arm. If the arm does not lock, repeat the release method and possibly **rock on your sacrum, and respiratory spinal extension** until your diaphragm becomes strong. Repeat as many times as needed.

CONTRAINDICATION

This method is NOT to be used on pregnant women. *(Refer to the Alternative Diaphragm Release Method— Rib Cage Release, on pg. 24.)*

DIAPHRAGM RELEASE

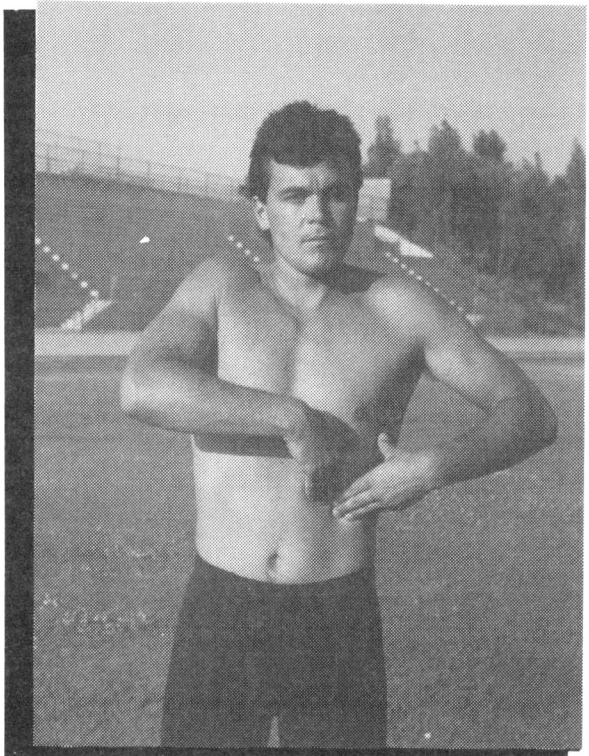

Figure A

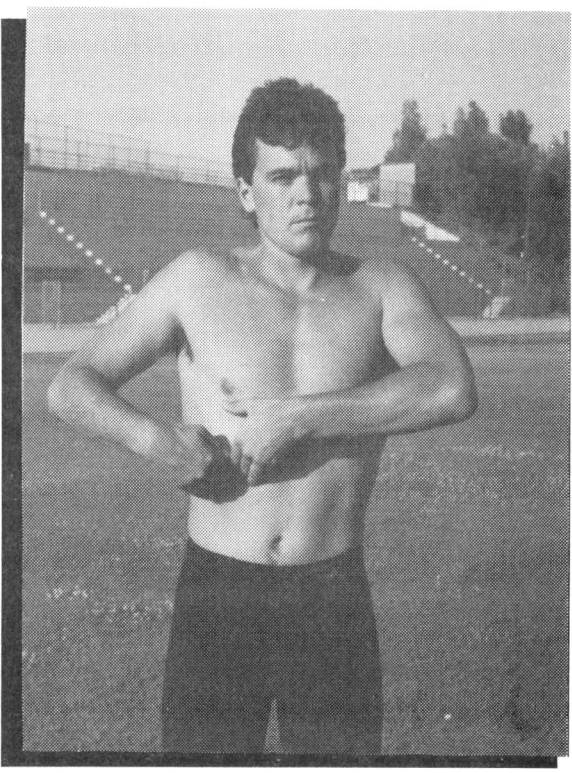

Figure C

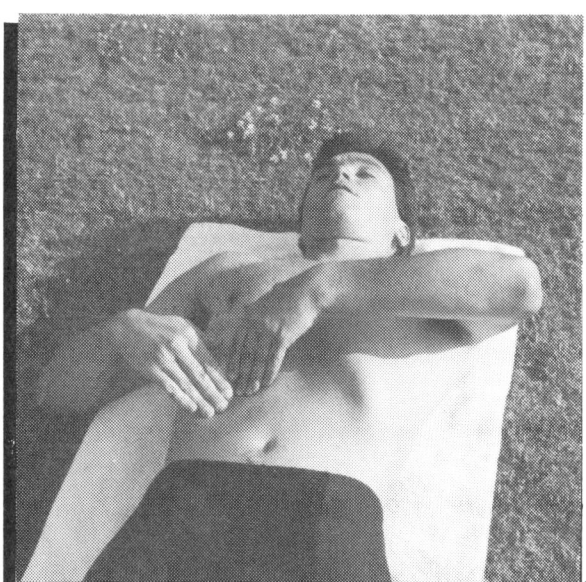

Figure B

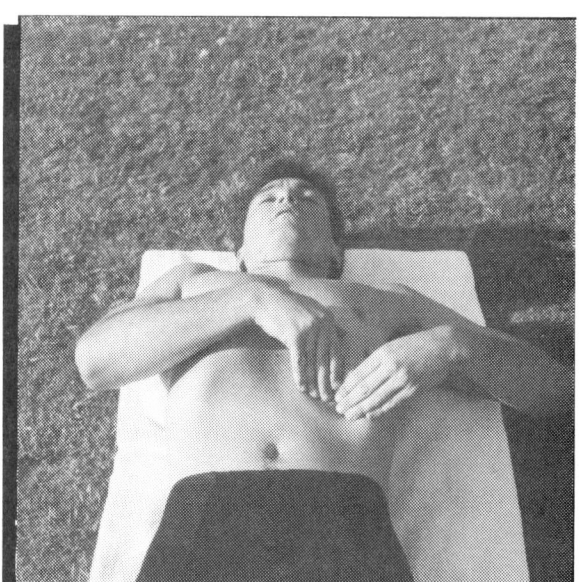

Figure D

ALTERNATIVE DIAPHRAGM RELEASE

RIB CAGE RELEASE

As pictured on pg. 25 standing or sitting, place hands on the side of the rib cage just below the breast area.

INHALE diaphragmatically, all the way up to your shoulders, exaggerating the lift in your shoulders, **hold your breath for an instant,** then **EXHALE** as you *gently but firmly* squeeze your rib cage to the full extent of your exhale. Repeat the process 3 times or as needed until you feel you have achieved a fuller and deeper breath. Continue to diaphragmatically breathe.

DIAPHRAGM RELEASE

ALTERNATIVE SELF-HELP METHOD (RIB CAGE RELEASE)

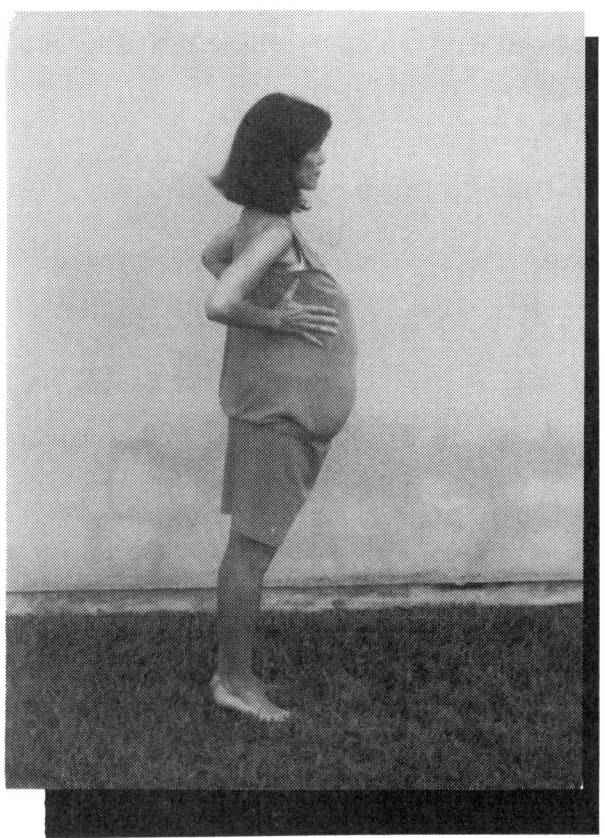

Susan Sparks

AUTONOMIC NERVOUS SYSTEM

In the **Autonomic Nervous System**, the nerves travel down along the spinal column and innervate the various organs and muscles of the body. These branches are known as plexus': The **solar plexus** innervates the diaphragm muscle via the vagus nerve. As the branch travels farther downward, it reaches the **sacral plexus**. If the sacrum is out of alignment and the diaphragm is inactive, the nerve pathway is disrupted. Both need to be functioning and in proper alignment to prevent short-circuiting of the body's energy system.

Based on experience with a wide spectrum of clients through teaching **diaphragmatic breathing, releasing a hypertonic diaphragm, rocking on the sacrum, and respiratory spinal extension for stretching the spine,** your energy can be properly reconnected producing a sense of revitalization.

(Pg. 27, gives a graphic illustration of the spinal plexus'.)

normal

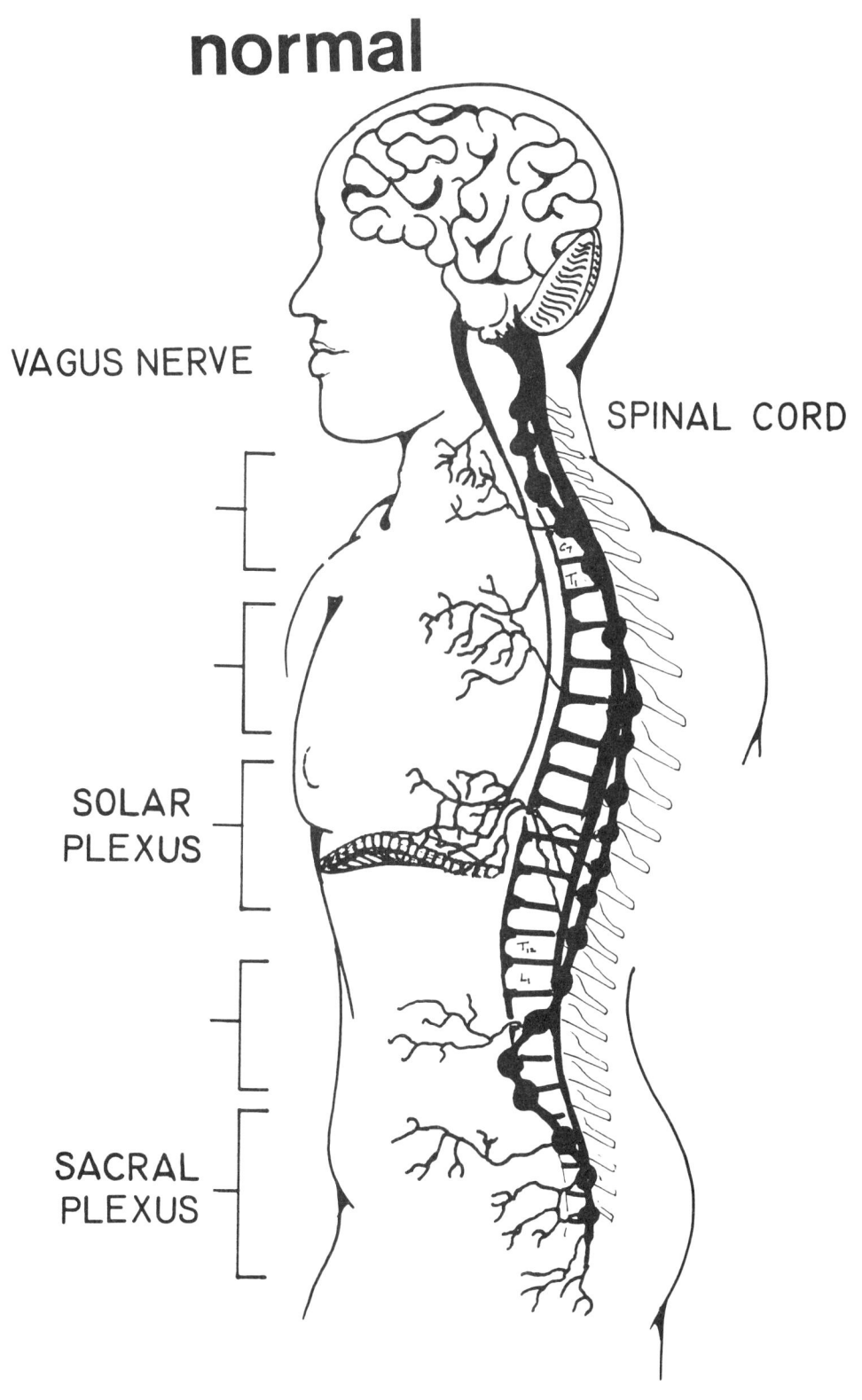

VAGUS NERVE

SPINAL CORD

SOLAR
PLEXUS

SACRAL
PLEXUS

Illustration by Greg Creswell

SACRAL MISALIGNMENT

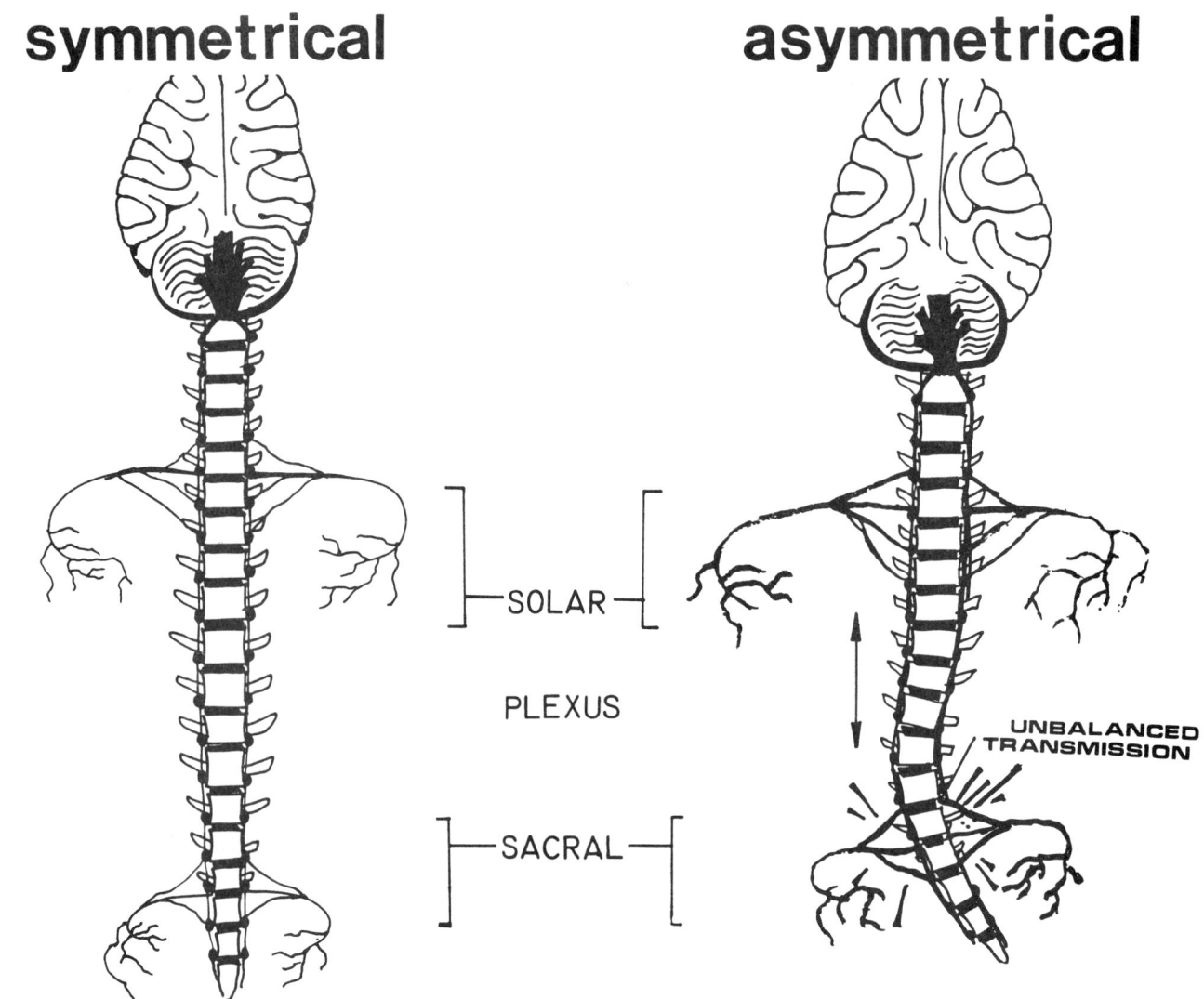

symmetrical   **asymmetrical**

SOLAR

PLEXUS

SACRAL

UNBALANCED TRANSMISSION

Illustration by Greg Creswell

SACRAL LIGAMENTS

Sacral Ligaments

Sacral Ligaments

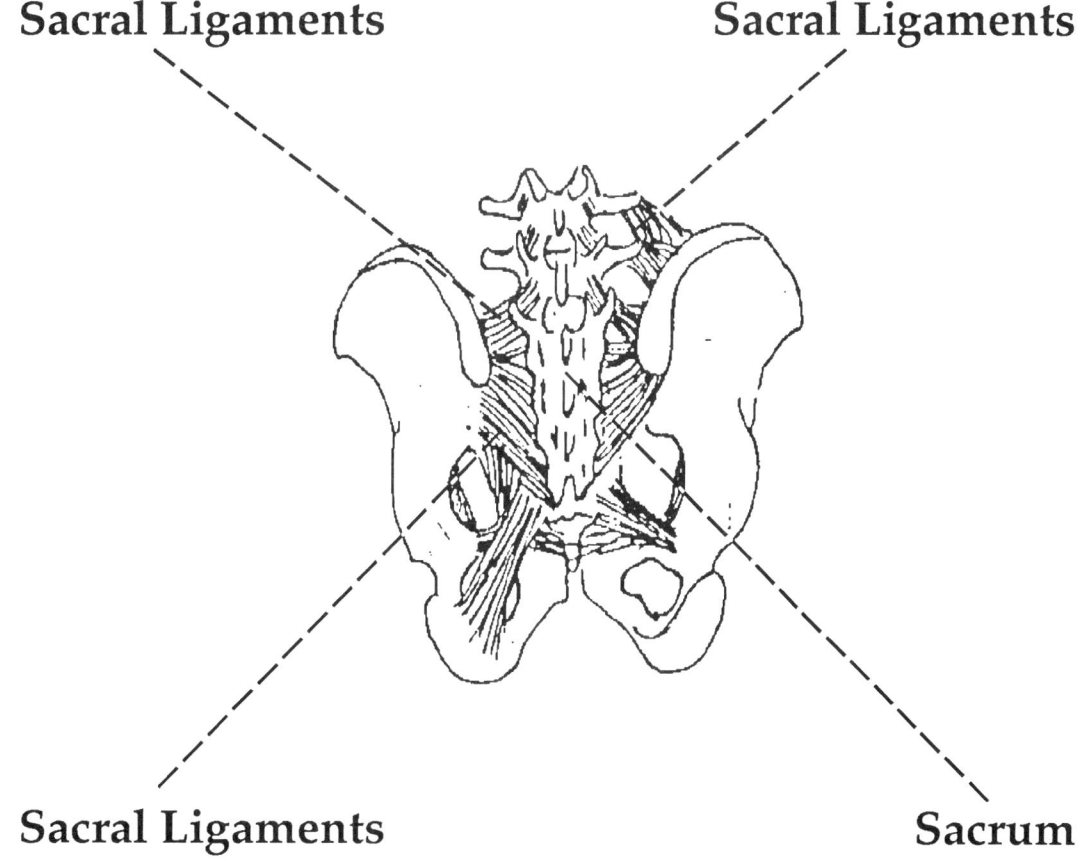

Sacral Ligaments

Sacrum

SACRAL ROCK
WHY WE "ROCK" ON THE SACRUM

The sacrum is located between the two ilium (hip bones) of the pelvis as pictured on pg. 29. It is held in place by tiny ligaments. When the sacral ligaments become stretched more to one side than the other, this can cause a shift in the sacrum creating a misalignment. (An example of this is sitting too much - secretary, long cycling trips, a truck driver, and most important, not diaphragmatically breathing.)

By sitting on a firm surface, placing your hands behind you for support, rock back and forth and side to side, you can stretch these ligaments. Thus moving the sacrum back into place.

The sacrum is also known as the "PUMP" for cerebral spinal fluid. By rocking on the sacrum you are pumping spinal fluid up and down the spine and into the brain. Spinal fluid is full of nutrients that keep the spine healthy and regenerated.

SACRAL ROCK

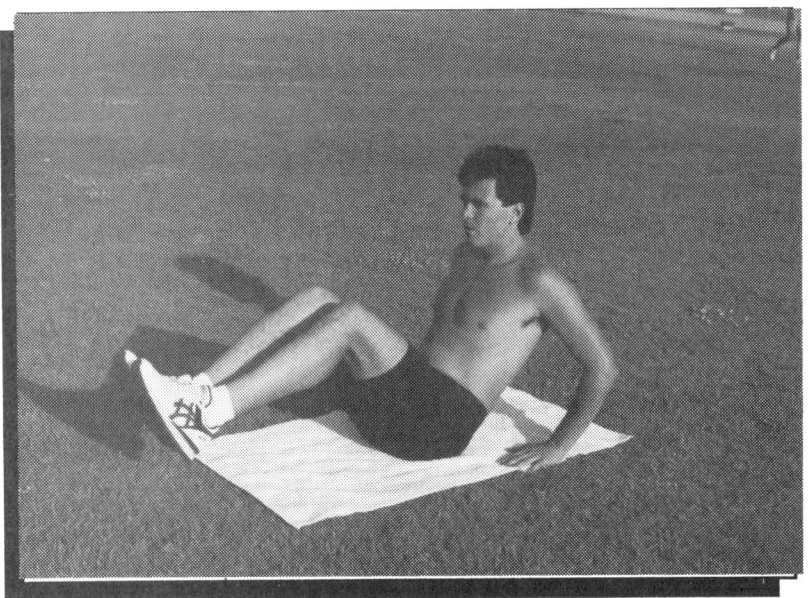

As pictured, sit on a hard padded surface with knees bent and raised. Rock front to back and side to side 3 times each direction. This movement stretches the ligaments of the sacrum and resets it so it is balanced between the two hipbones.

Figure A

FRONT TO BACK ROCK

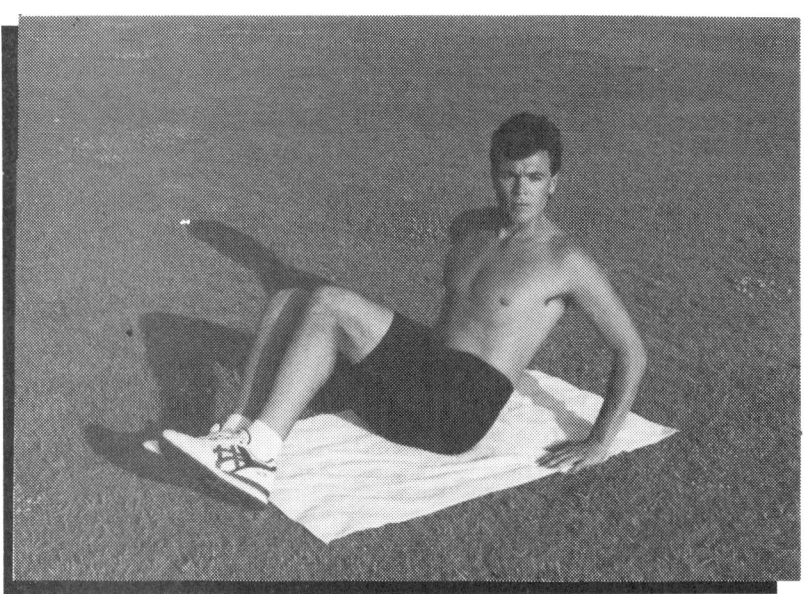

Figure B

SIDE TO SIDE ROCK

RESPIRATORY SPINAL EXTENSION

As pictured, on pg. 33, lie on your side with bottom shoulder out from under you, keeping your bottom leg straight.

INHALE diaphragmatically, and as you EXHALE, grasp the knee of the upper leg and pull toward your opposite shoulder. Do this on each side or as many times as necessary.

This action helps to release the sacrum, allowing greater extension of the legs. It also creates a stretch for the spinal muscles of the back, easing tensions throughout the entire spine.

RESPIRATORY SPINAL EXTENSION

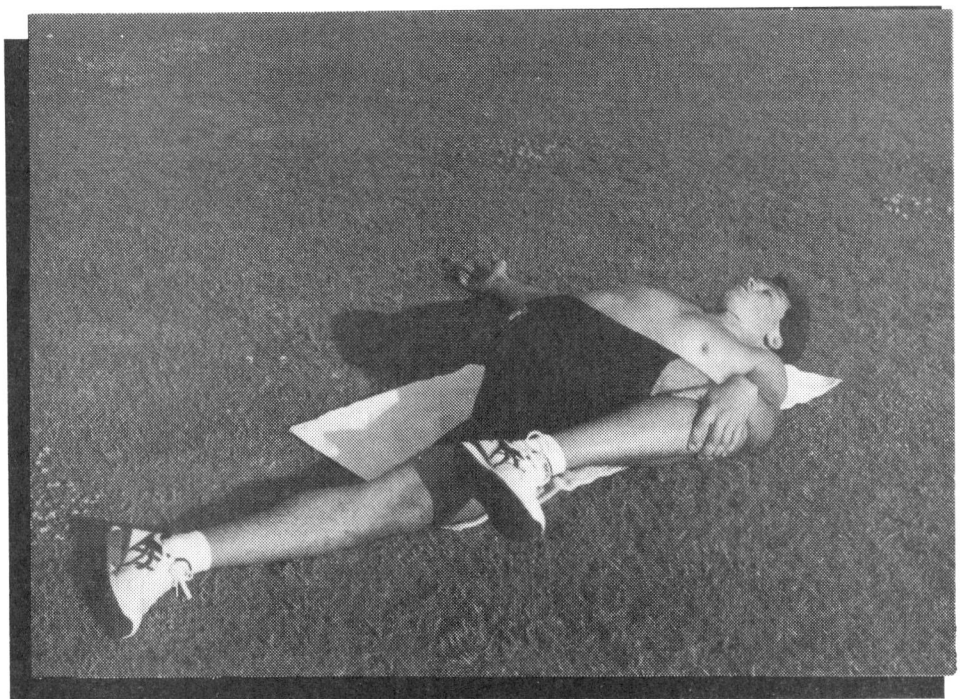

Figure A

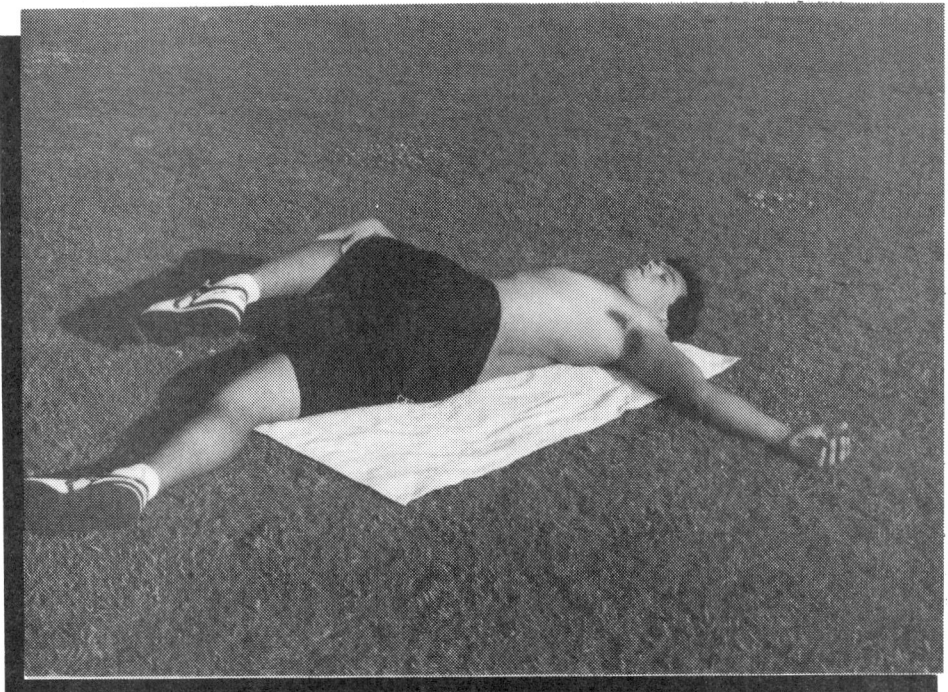

Figure B

THE ATHLETE

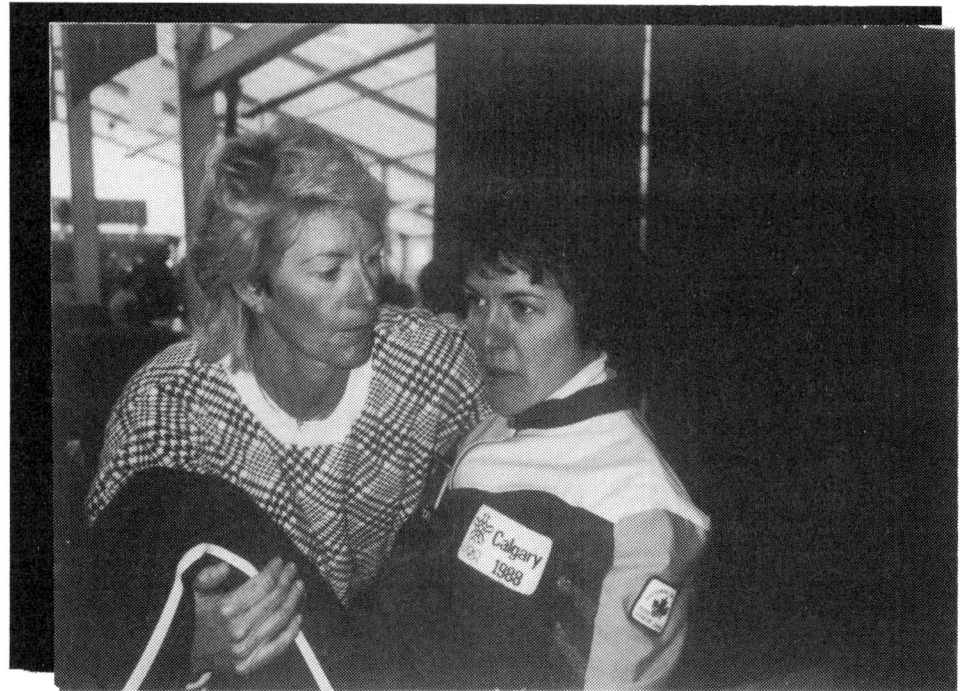

Sacral Rock

"Thanks to Kate and her muscle balancing techniques, plus her pre-event massage before my race, I was so energized! I was able to compete in my final day of competition without feeling totally exhausted."

Angela Schmidt-Foster
1988 Canadian Olympic
Cross-Country Ski Team
Calgary, Alberta, Canada

TWO–MINUTE ENERGY BALANCE

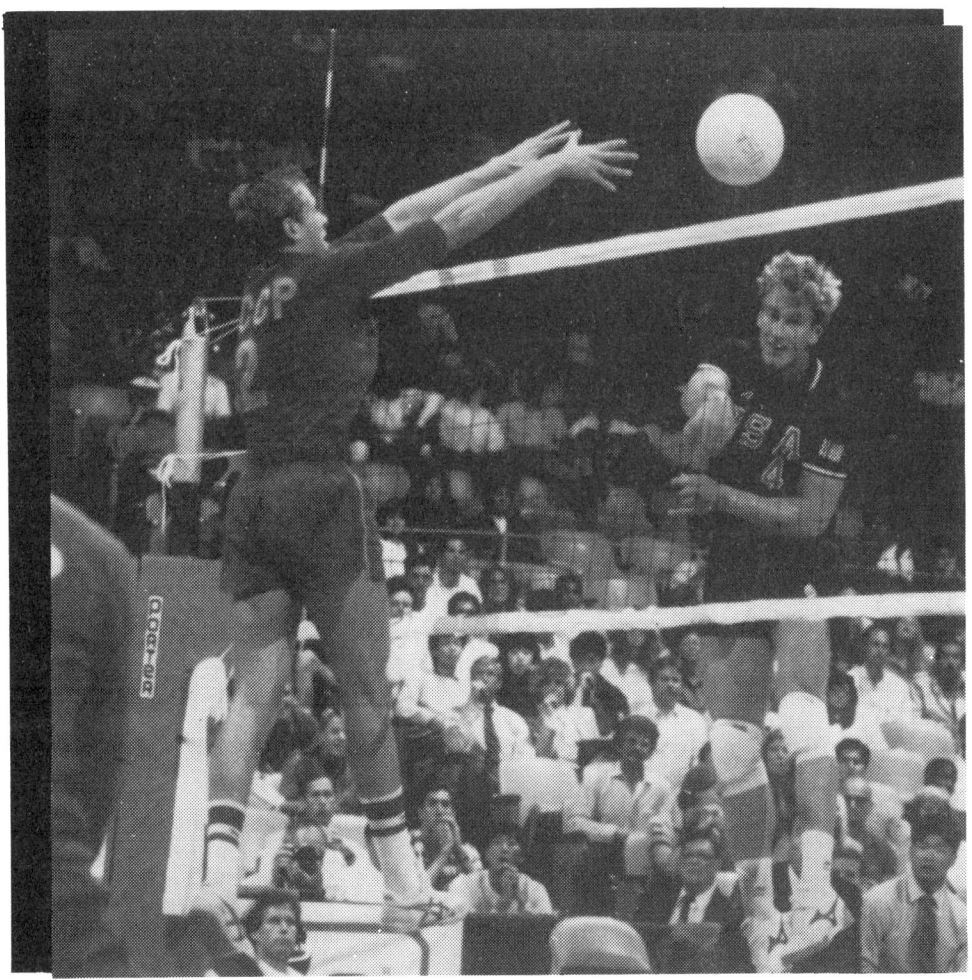

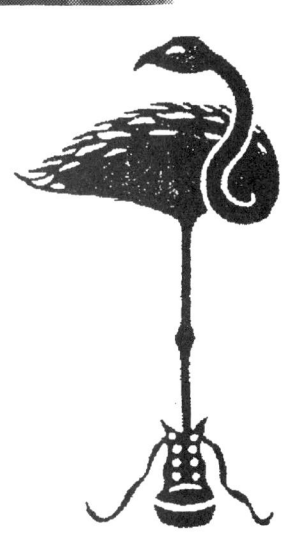

"I don't do the Ritual everyday, but when I'm preparing for lesser meets I do a few of the steps just to give me an edge. Then when I'm in major competitions, I do the complete Ritual to get myself totally balanced and ready. My body feels revitalized and primed for action!"

Bob Ctvrtlik

1988 USA Volleyball Team
Gold Medal Winner
Seoul Olympic Games

IMMUNE SYSTEM

The human immune system is an amazingly intricate biochemical network which arms us against enemies such as cold viruses, to bacterial infections and cancer. Unfortunately, the effects of stress in our daily lives have a direct bearing on how efficiently our immune system works. Its delicate balance can be upset by a variety of factors.

When the "vital energy" of the body is challenged due to emotional stress, lack of exercise, poor nutrition, insufficient sleep or indulgences of coffee, alcohol, drugs or cigarettes, your energy balance either wanes or becomes over-activated.

When these stressors cause our immune system to become under active, we feel sluggish and fatigued; when over-activated, we experience anxiety and a sense of being pressured or "stressed out." Either condition creates imbalances of vital energy in our organs of detoxification — The liver, kidneys, and spleen. When these organs are "out-of-balance" our water intake may be off, elimination process clogged, and all our biochemical processes function below par. For example, eating too much sugar will cause the adrenal glands to work overtime, thus creating a need for our pancreas to over compensate, which throws our entire system off kilter.

With so many stress factors in our daily lives — some avoidable, others not — it's vitally important to keep our immune system strong enough to handle a constant stream of challenge.

By getting up each morning and performing a simple ritual called the "Two-Minute Energy Balance," you can help maintain your body's vital energy, and thus maximize the stability of your immune system.

To determine your current energy level, **firmly rub the Energy Barometer, C.V. 17**, pictured on pg. 51. If you experience soreness, it means that energy is not flowing fluidly throughout your body and your emotions are being "stuffed" or put on hold. When your body is functioning as it should, *this point should never be sore*.

To strengthen the vital energy, drain poisons and toxins from the body, while enhancing athletic ability and coordination, perform the **Two-Minute Energy Balance daily** to keep your body strong and healthy.

TWO MINUTE ENERGY BALANCE

Begin by standing. Do the following:

I.   Diaphragmatically breathe 10 times.

II.   Release the diaphragm muscle.

III. Sacral Rock 3 times each direction, back and forth and side to side.

IV.   Respiratory Spinal Extension.

BODY ENERGY BALANCING

I.   Neuro-logical Integration: Rub the top of the coccyx (tailbone) Governing Vessel 2 and naval in a clockwise, circular motion for 20 seconds, (long version), 10 seconds, (short version). Use medium to firm pressure. (Pg.. 39)

PURPOSE: To balance all the body's chemistry and center the body's awareness toward health.

Governing Vessel 2 - centers the body's awareness toward good health.

Naval - 12 meridians meet here. Circling clockwise will balance all the body's chemistry.

BENEFITS: To create good health with positive thoughts and intent.

II.   Neuro-logical Integration: Rub the top of the coccyx (tailbone) Governing Vessel 2 and right Kidney 27 simultaneously for 20 seconds, (long version), 10 seconds, (short version). Use medium to firm pressure. (Pg. 39)

PURPOSE: To drain lymphatics of the lower third of the spinal cord and to get rid of swelling (edema) that can cause pain. If severe low back pain arises, rub 3 minutes to drain the toxins and poisons that contribute to low back pain.

BENEFITS: Increased flexibility and movement of the lower back.

III. Neuro-logical Integration: Now rub top of coccyx (tailbone) Governing Vessel 2 and left Kidney 27 simultaneously for 20 seconds, (long version), 10 seconds, (short version). Use medium to firm pressure. (Pg. 39)

PURPOSE: To drain the lymphatics of the whole spinal cord and drain the toxins and poisons that contribute to back pain, and to get rid of swelling (edema) that can cause pain.

BENEFITS: Increased flexibility and movement of the whole spine. (Example: neck and shoulder pain.)

TWO MINUTE ENERGY BALANCE

IV. Switch-board Turn-on: Place thumb and index finger of right hand on Kidney 27 points located at the end of the clavicle (collarbone) on each side of the sternum. Rub firmly, in a pinching motion, while the left hand rests on the naval. Repeat action with hands reversed, 30 seconds each hand, (long version), 10 seconds each hand, (short version). (Pg. 41)

PURPOSE: To fully organize the integrity of the neural system of the body for better coordination.

BENEFITS: Better athletic ability and coordination, which involves better sight, dexterity, hearing and alertness.

V. Balancing the meridian energy of the front and back of the body:

Front: Lightly hold Conception Vessel 2, located at the top of the Pubis, midline and Conception Vessel 24, located in the depression above the chin and below the lower lip, for 30 seconds, (long version), 10 seconds, (short version), breathing steadily. (Pg. 42)

Back: Lightly hold Governing Vessel 2, located at the top of the coccyx (tailbone), and Governing Vessel 26, located midline above the upper lip, under the nose, for 30 seconds, (long version), 10 seconds, (short version), breathing steadily. (Pg. 42)

PURPOSE: To enhance coordination and alertness between the front and back of the body. (Example: The right hand knows what the left hand is doing.)

BENEFITS: Better athletic agility and coordination, which involves better sight, dexterity, hearing and alertness.

VI. Neuro-Muscular Integration: By performing marching patterns such as Cross Crawl and Homo-lateral, this further integrates the body/mind. (Pg 44)

PURPOSE: To provide better coordination and agility for an athlete.

BENEFITS: Increased sight, dexterity, hearing, alertness, and sharpness of mind/body.

NEURO-LOGICAL INTEGRATION

Balancing Energy Diagram I, II, III

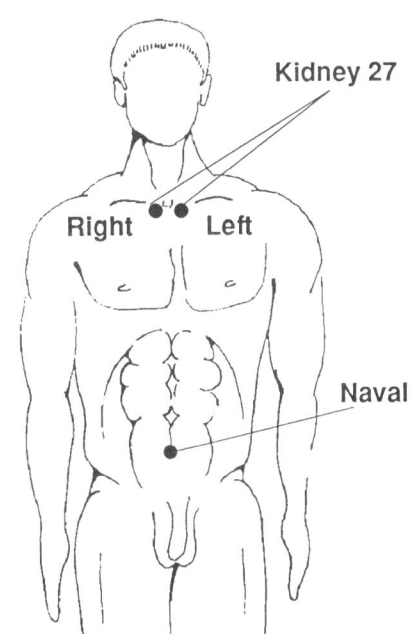

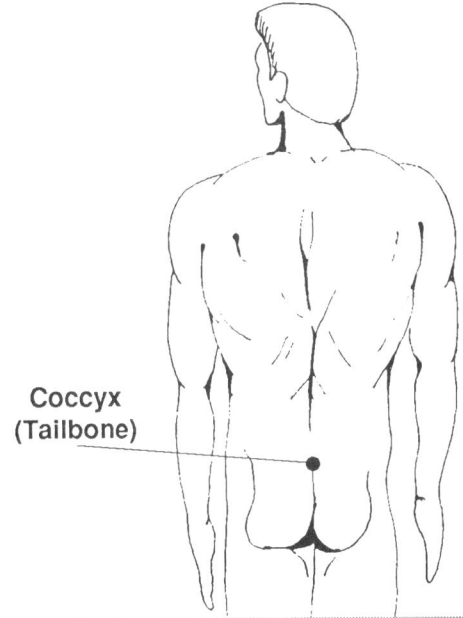

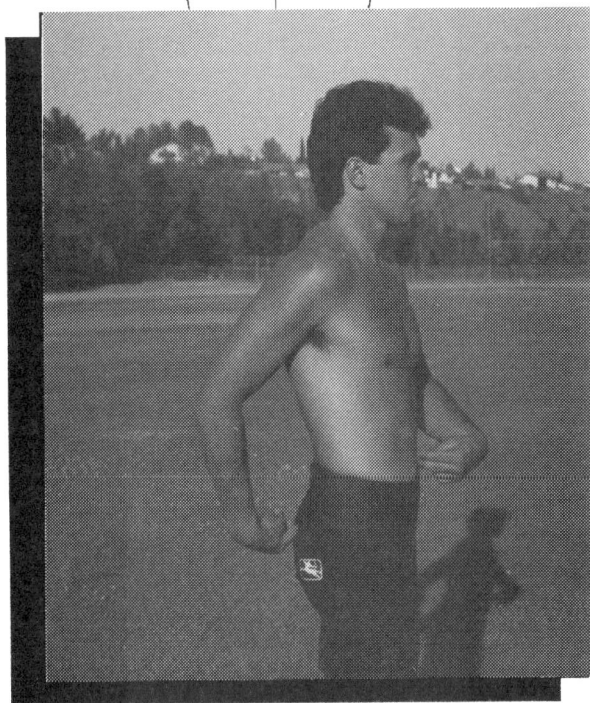

Rub top of coccyx and rub naval clockwise simultaneously for 20 seconds. Purpose is to balance the body's chemistry and center the body's awareness toward health. Opens the channels to neuro-integration.

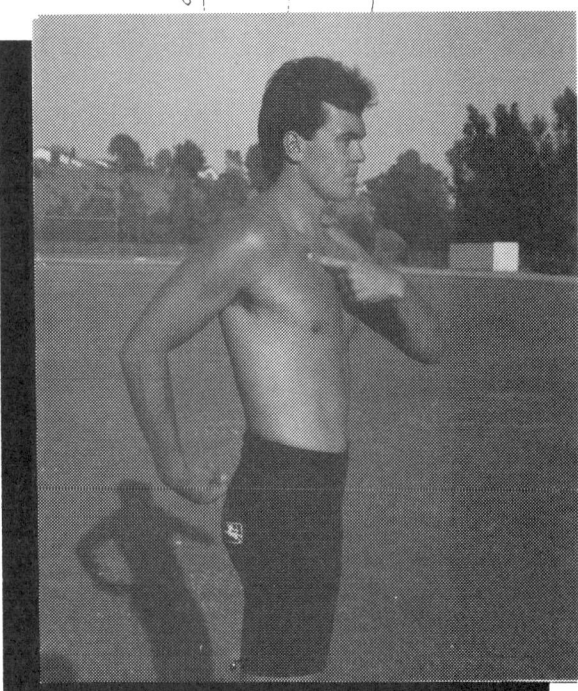

Rub top of coccyx G.V. 2 and and right kidney 27 simultaneously for 20 seconds. (If severe low-back pain, rub 3 minutes.) Drains lymphatic vessels of lower one-third of spinal cord. Now rub coccyx G.V. 2 and left kidney 27 simultaneously for 20 seconds. Drains all the lymphatic vessels of the spinal cord.

SWITCHING

"**Switching**" is a phenomenom in the neural system that reverses the nerves' pathway between the right brain and the left brain. The normal situation is to have the left brain direct impulses to the right side of the body, and the right brain direct impulses to the left side of the body. Your left brain is your logical, analytical side and the right brain is your creative, feeling side. When the nerve impulses become "switched," this causes mental and physical confusion and lack of agility and coordination. This can be caused by emotional upset, trauma to the body, and stress of any kind, and overworked muscles that have been pushed beyond their capabilities.

When the body is fully organized, athletic endurance and agility are enhanced. The **Switchboard Turn-on** (pg. 41) helps correct energy switching in the body. The integrity of the neural system leads to better coordination and overall ability of the athlete.

ACUPRESSURE BODY ORGANIZATION
SWITCHBOARD TURN-ON
Balancing Energy Diagram IV

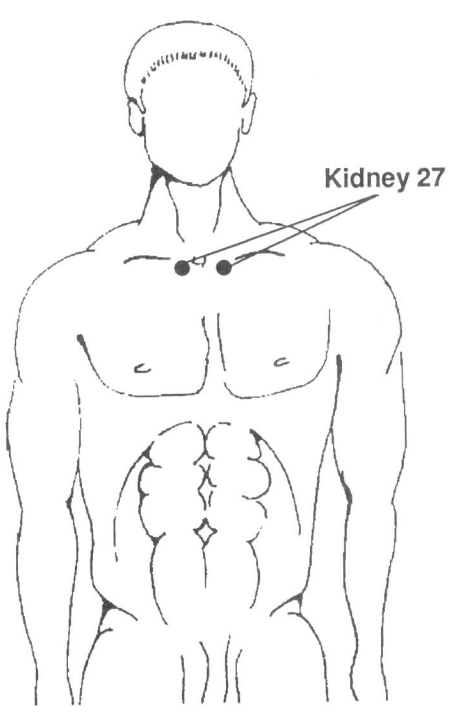

Kidney 27

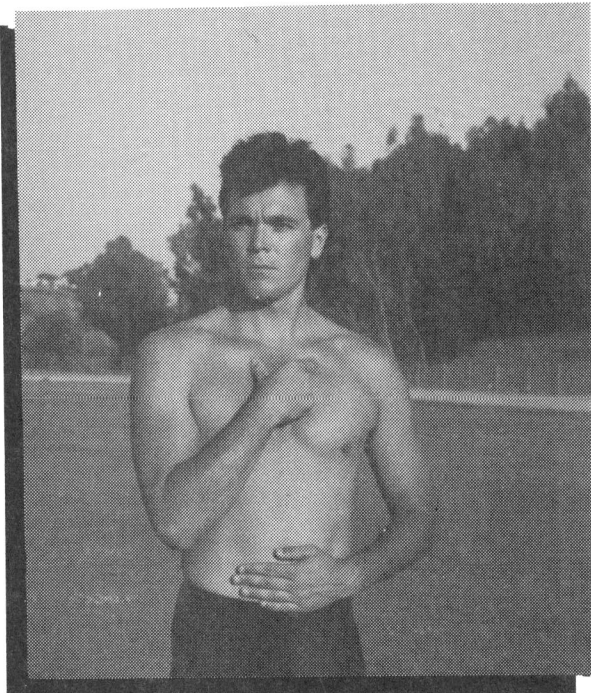

Figure 5A

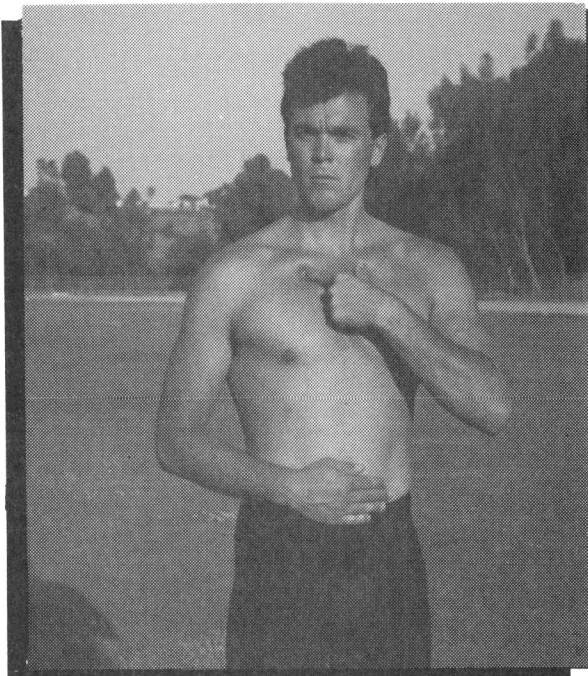

Figure 5B

Place thumb and index finger of right hand on Kidney 27 points (indentations), located at the end of the clavicle (collarbone) on each side of sternum and rub firmly in a pinching motion while left hand rests on navel. Repeat action with hands reversed, 30 seconds each hand.

Illustration by Greg Creswell

BALANCING MERIDIAN ENERGY

Balancing Energy Diagram V

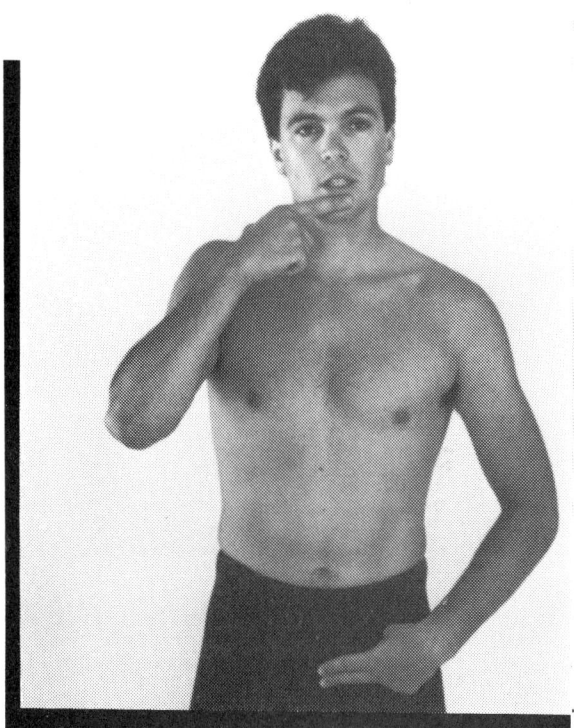

Proper balance is essential for success in any athletic endeavor. Muscles become sore from overuse. The body adjusts to relieve soreness — often throwing the body's energy systems out of balance. Holding these points enhances coordination and alertness between the front and back of the body.

FRONT

Figure A

Lightly hold Conception Vessel 2 located midline at the top of the Pubis and Conception Vessel 24 located in the depression above the chin and below the lower lip for 30 seconds - breathing steadily.

BACK

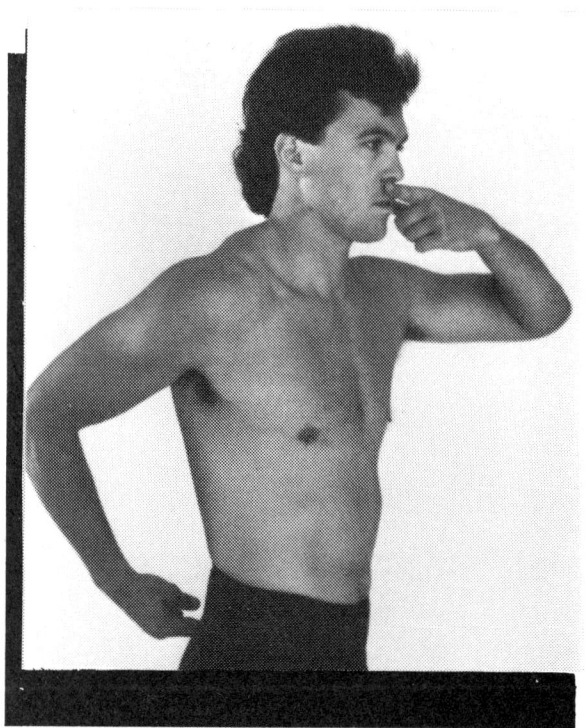

Figure B

Lightly hold Governing Vessel 2 located at the top of the Coccyx and Governing Vessel 26 located below the nose and above the upper lip for 30 seconds - breathing steadily.

BALANCING MERIDIAN ENERGY

Balancing Energy Diagram Step V

Front and Back Body Energy

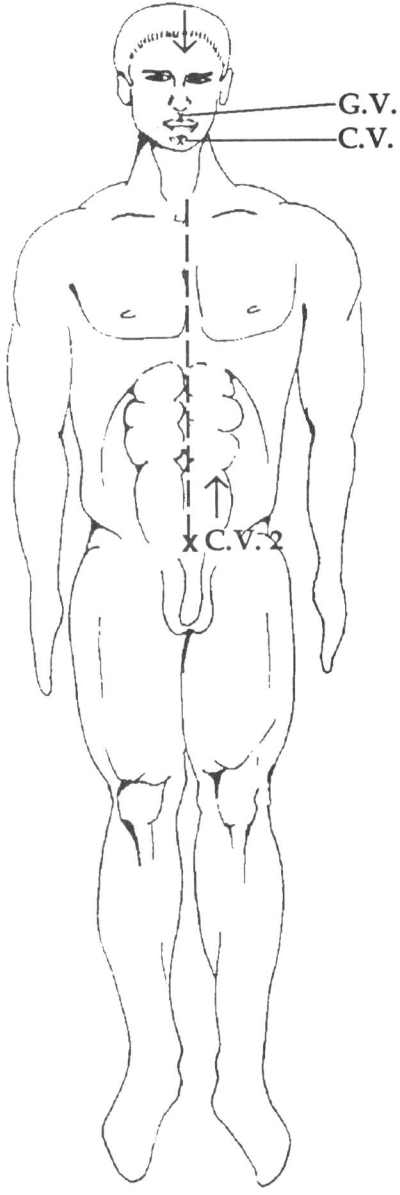

G.V. 26
C.V. 24

x C.V. 2

Conception Vessel Meridian

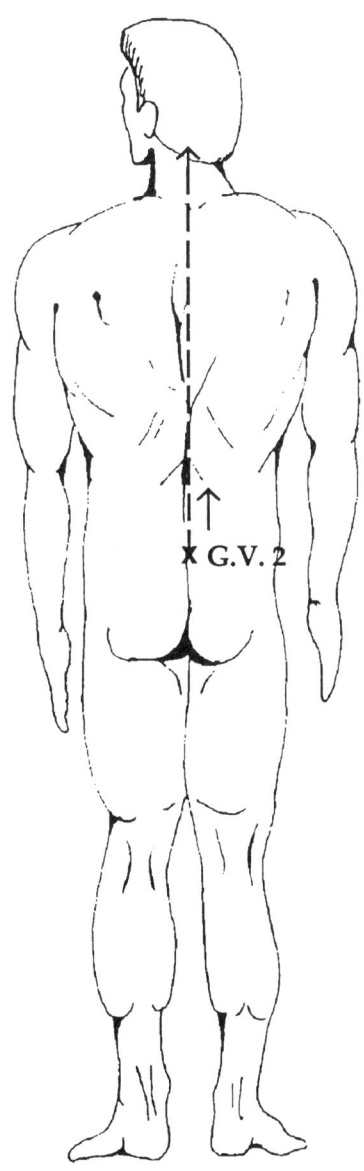

x G.V. 2

Governing Vessel Meridian

Illustration by Greg Creswell

NEURO-MUSCULAR INTEGRATION

Balancing Energy Diagram VI

Cross-Crawl Pattern
March in place as pictured on far left. Move your right arm to your left knee and left arm to right. At the same time move your eyes right to left and up and down. Open and close your eyes.

Homolateral Pattern
Switch and march, touching your right arm to your right knee and your left arm to your left knee. Move your eyes right, left, up, down and open and close them.

Do both patterns until the transitions are easy and fluid.

These patterns help to Force-Feed activities into as many parts of the brain as possible.

Always end with a Cross-Crawl.

Advanced Marching Pattern
March in place. Count from 2-4-6-8-10 to 100, while moving eyes clockwise then counter-clockwise. Repeat this pattern with eyes closed. This integrates the left brain.

While marching begin to hum repeating the movements of the eyes clockwise, counter-clockwise and with eyes closed. This integrates the right brain.

For further integration, move your head right to left while doing cross crawl marching.

The advanced patterns only need to be done in Cross-Crawl pattern. All patterns should be done in an easy free-flowing movement.

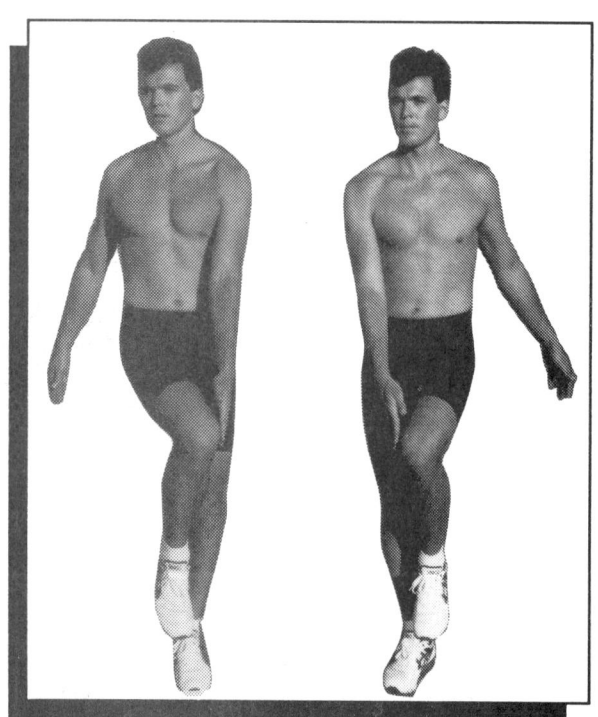

Cross-Crawl Pattern

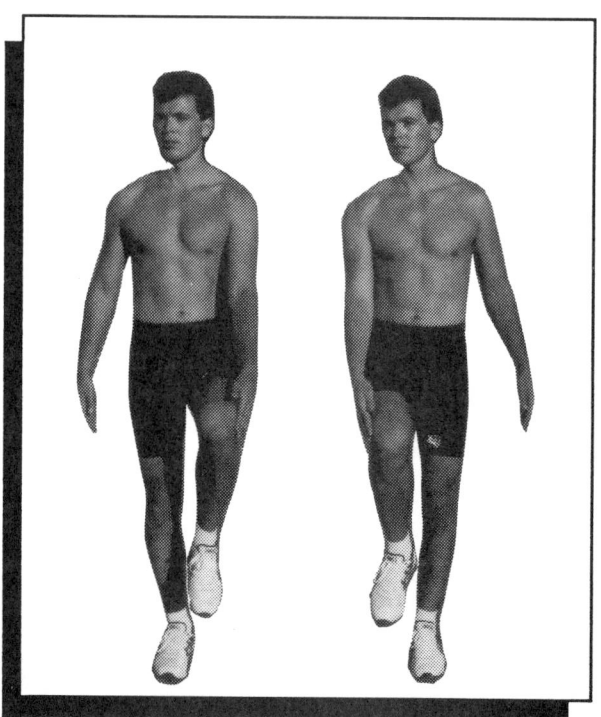

Homolateral Pattern

ACUPRESSURE
FOR INCREASED ENERGY AND PERFORMANCE

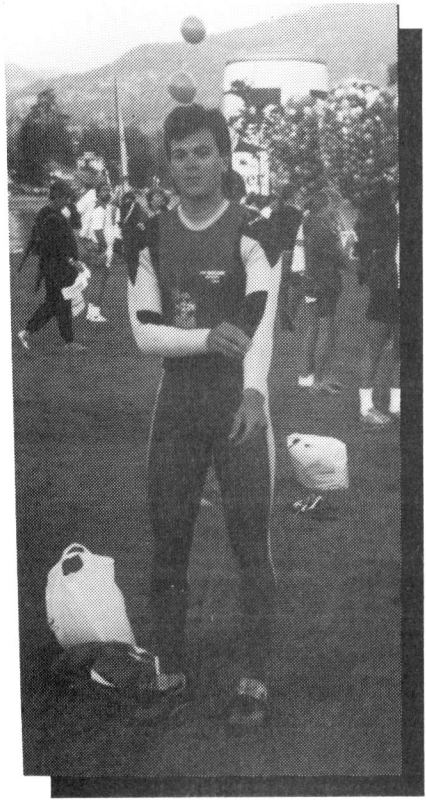

David Hemingway

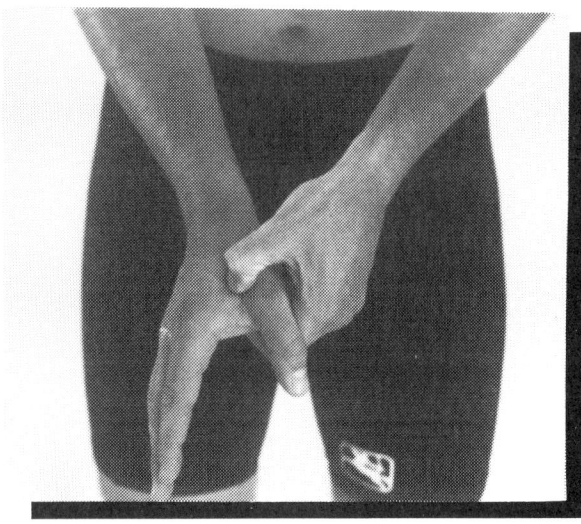

"Techniques of Oriental Medicine have long been used as a means to treat and prevent disease, enhance health and vitality. The modern application of these techniques in working with athletes is an appropriate extension of the Therapeutic effect long verified by the practical use of Acupuncture.

"World-class sports trainers from around the globe have practitioners of Acupuncture/acupressure and massage as part of their training teams. Their presence plays an important role in performance and recovery.

"The information put forth in this book can assist athletes at all levels to utilize the health enhancing benefits of Oriental Medicine."

Richard M. Gold, PhD.,C.A.
Licensed Acupuncturist

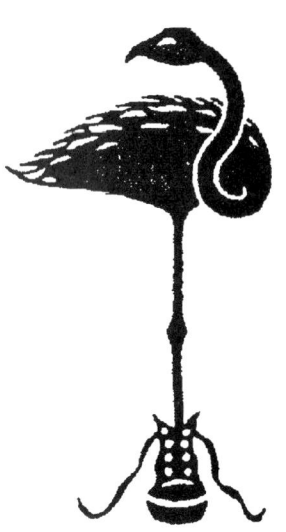

ACUPRESSURE

Traditional Chinese Medicine has been in existence for many centuries. However, the use of Acupuncture in this country is just now becoming recognized as a viable form of medical treatment.

Acupressure, a non-invasive form of Acupuncture, is practiced by applying pressure at points along the fourteen meridian channels. By pressing on these points, it is possible to release "**Blocked Energy**", which can then flow fluidly throughout the body to relieve pain, muscle soreness, headaches, and a variety of other disorders. Each meridian channel is associated with a particular vital organ and muscle in the body.

Both **Acupressure** and **Acupuncture** can effectively eliminate or reduce numerous acute as well as chronic problems associated with disabling aches and pains.

I teach **Acupressure points** to the athletes as an additional tool they can use during warm-up and cool-down and for maintenance of their vital energy, stamina, endurance and overall health.

ACUPRESSURE FOR INCREASED ENERGY AND PERFORMANCE

Go Points

1. Large Intestine 4: Moves blood and Qi.
2. Large Intestine 10: Stimulates the Adrenals.
3. Stomach 36: Increases Vitality.
4. Triple Warmer 4: Raises the Yang, Energy.
5. Conception Vessel 12: Yang organs meet here.
6. Conception Vessel 17: Releases the Qi, Emotions, and aids in respiration. Used as an indicator, barometer, of a person's energy.

Cool Down Points

1. Spleen 6: Builds the Yin.
2. Heart 7: "Shenmen", relaxes the muscles.
3. Conception Vessel 4: Energy of the Kidneys meets here. Lay hands over the lower abdomen.
4. Urinary Bladder 23/Gallbladder 25: Lay hands over the back where the Kidneys are located.

Competition Points

1. Kidney 3: Focusing.
2. Large Intestine 10: Stimulates the Adrenals.
3. Stomach 36: Increases Vitality.
4. Conception Vessel 17: Releases the Qi, Emotions, and aids in respiration.

Immune System

1. Large Intestine 11/Large Intestine 4/Spleen 6/Stomach 36: Stimulates.
2. Large Intestine 11/Stomach 36: Used together to move energy "Qi". (These points are good to use to heal an injury).

ACUPRESSURE FOR INCREASED ENERGY AND PERFORMANCE

Associated Points Relating to Symptoms

1. Spleen 3: Sugar, Corresponding muscle -- Latissimus Dorsi.
2. Kidney 3: Salt, Dehydration -- Psoas.
3. Stomach 36/Kidney 27: Stamina and Balance.
4. Large Intestine 4/Liver 3/Triple Warmer 23: Headache.
5. Conception Vessel 12: Digestion.
6. Large Intestine 4/Liver 3/Heart 7/Conception Vessel 12: Jet Lag. Spleen 21 and pull ears in all directions.

* To stimulate a point, such as for the Go, Competitive, Immune System -- **Pump firmly** on the point 10 times.

* To sedate, such as for the Cool Down Points, simply **hold the point** *gently*.

Acupressure Abbreviations Used

Large Intestine ....Lg. I.

Stomach ....St.

Triple Warmer ......................................T.W.

Conception Vessel ......................................C.V.

Spleen ....Sp.

Heart ....Ht.

Urinary Bladder ......................................U.B.

Gall Bladder......................................G.B.

Kidney ....K.

Liver......................................Li.

ACUPRESSURE GO POINTS

TO MOVE ENERGY AND BLOOD:

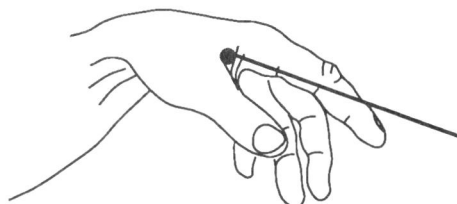

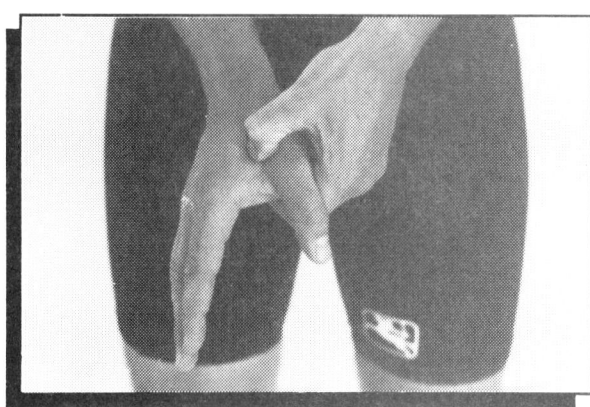

Large Intestine 4 Located between 1st and 2nd metacarpal bones, in the crease between the two fingers. Locate point and **pump firmly** 10 times.

TO STIMULATE ADRENALS:

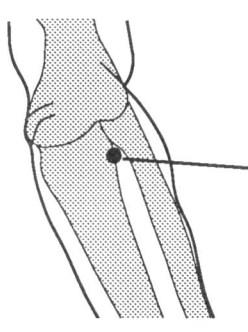

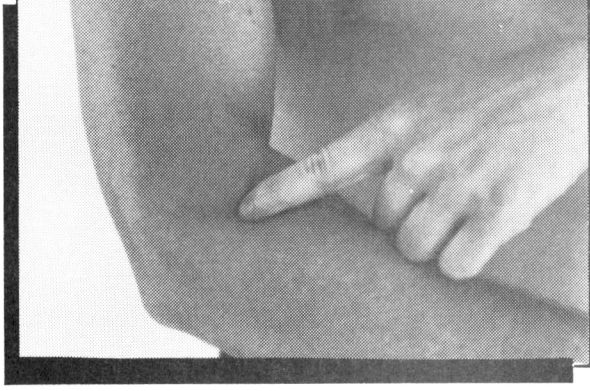

Large Intestine 10 Located two fingers below the crease of the elbow. With palm down, locate point and **pump firmly** 10 times.

TO INCREASE VITALITY:

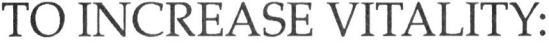

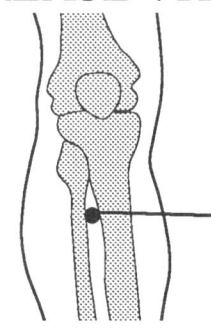

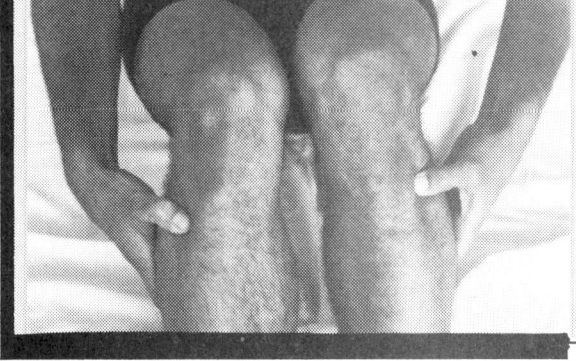

Stomach 36 Slide finger up Tibialis Anterior muscle to the depression before the head of the tibia. **Pump firmly** 10 times.

Illustrations by Judy Smith

ACUPRESSURE COOL DOWN POINTS

Vascular points appear to improve circulation to muscles and organs increasing their strength. The forehead points relate to digestive function and brain function.

TO RELIEVE EMOTIONAL STRAIN:

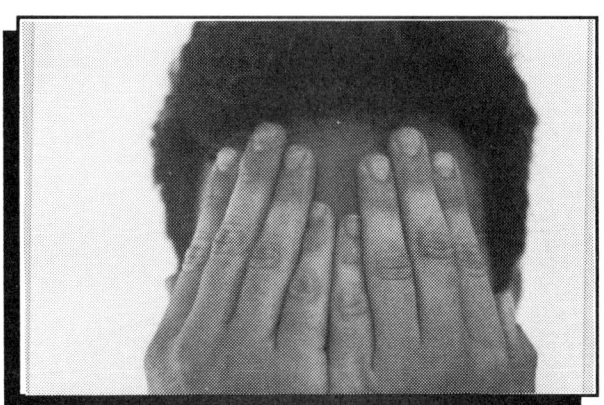

Place fingertips on middle of forehead. Press and hold for 30-60 seconds or until you are calmer and your mind clears.

TO DECREASE STRESS ON THE KIDNEYS:

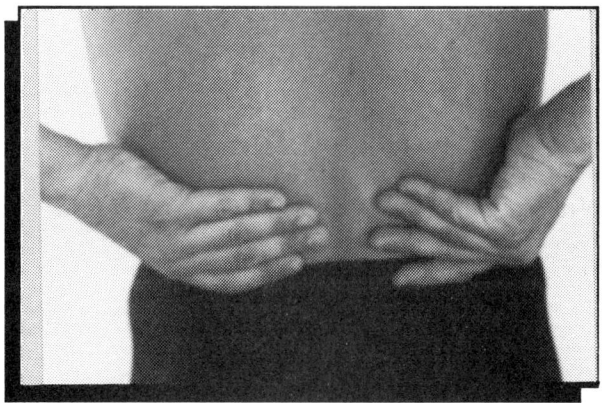

Hold hands over kidneys 30 to 60 seconds. Drink plenty of water.

TO RELAX MUSCLES AND TENSIONS FROM THE BODY:

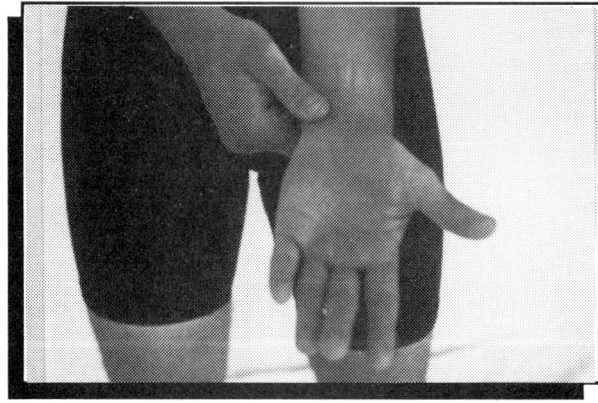

Heart 7 Place thumb just below the Pisiform Bone (little finger side) on the wrist. Hold lightly for 30-60 seconds.

ACUPRESSURE
BODY ENERGY BAROMETER

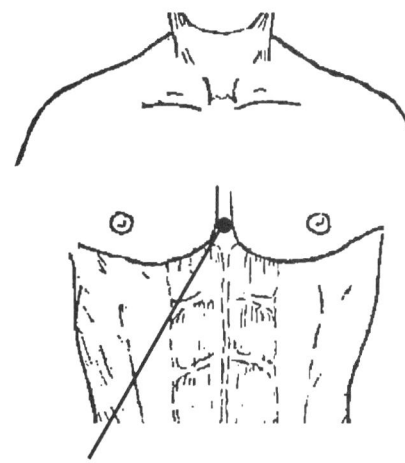

Conception Vessel 17 Firmly rubbing the pressure point on the sternum directly between the nipples helps to disperse energy throughout the body. This point tells you if your energy is blocked or not. It should never be sore. Soreness means blocked energy.

Rub firmly 30 seconds.

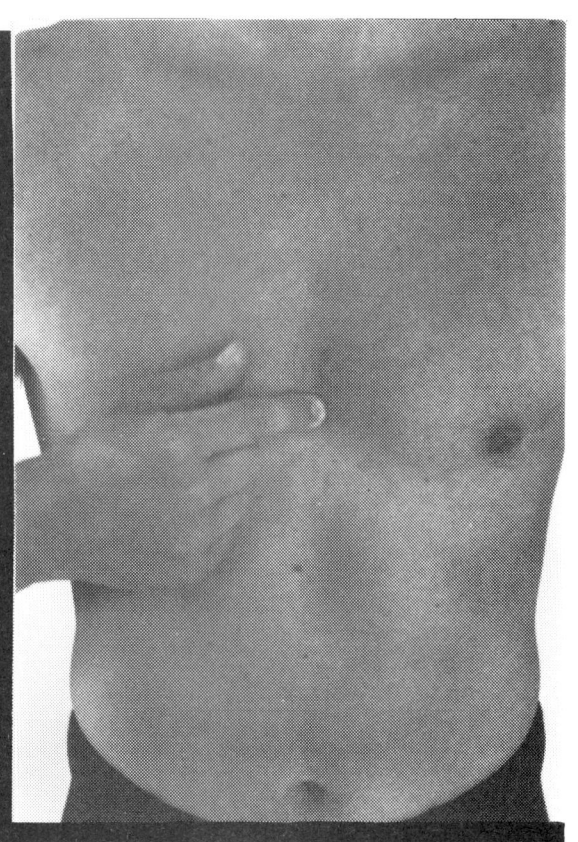

Illustration by Judy Smith

ACUPRESSURE FOR INCREASED ENERGY AND PERFORMANCE

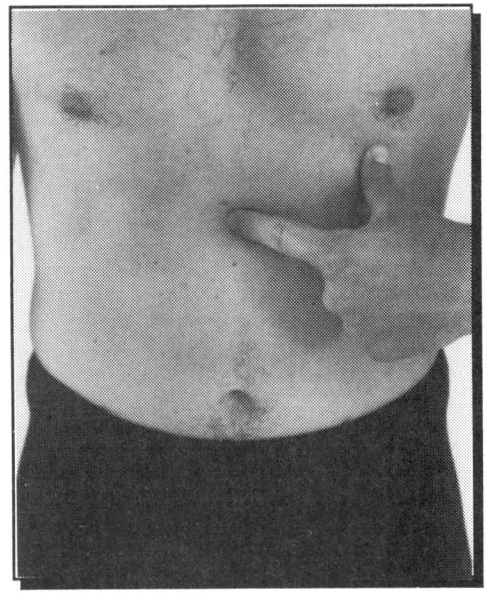

C.V. 12
- *"Jet Lag"*
- *Digestion*

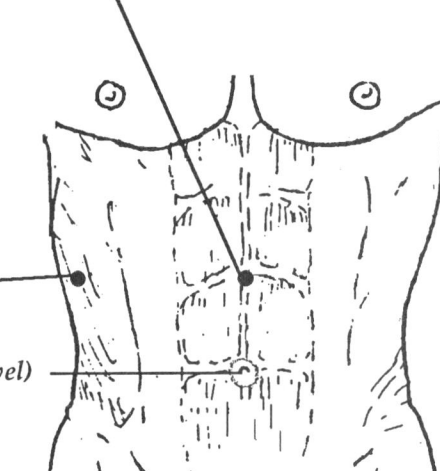

SPL. 21
- *"Jet Lag"*

(Navel)

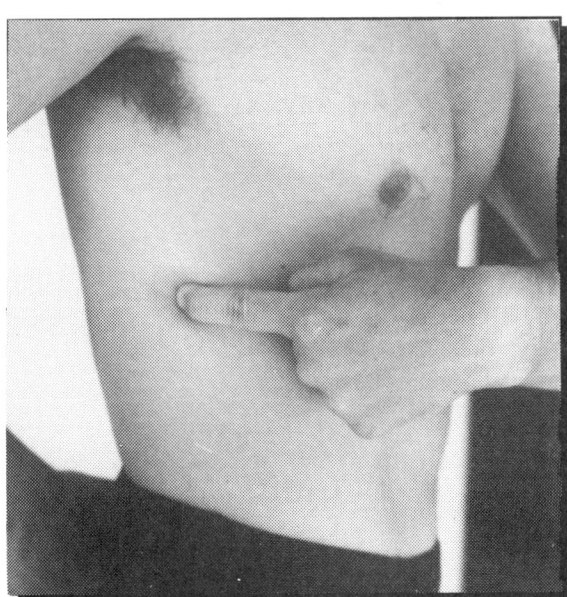

C.V. 4
- *Kidney Energy*

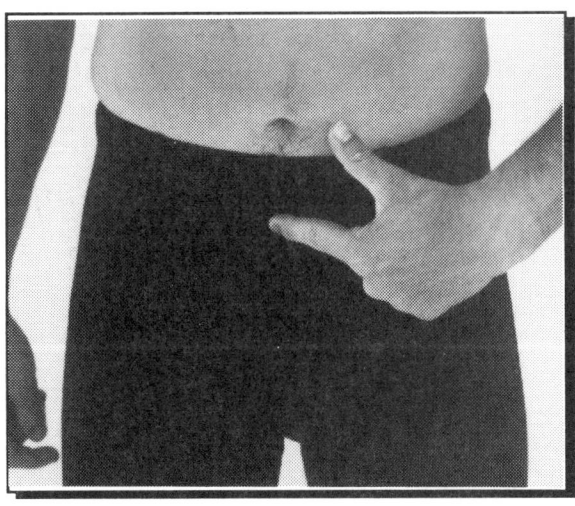

Illustrations by Judy Smith

ACUPRESSURE FOR INCREASED ENERGY AND PERFORMANCE

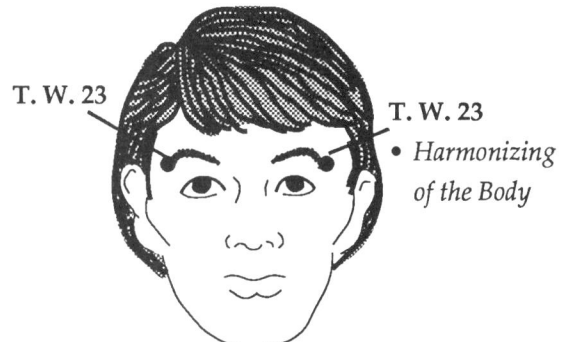

T. W. 23

T. W. 23
• *Harmonizing of the Body*

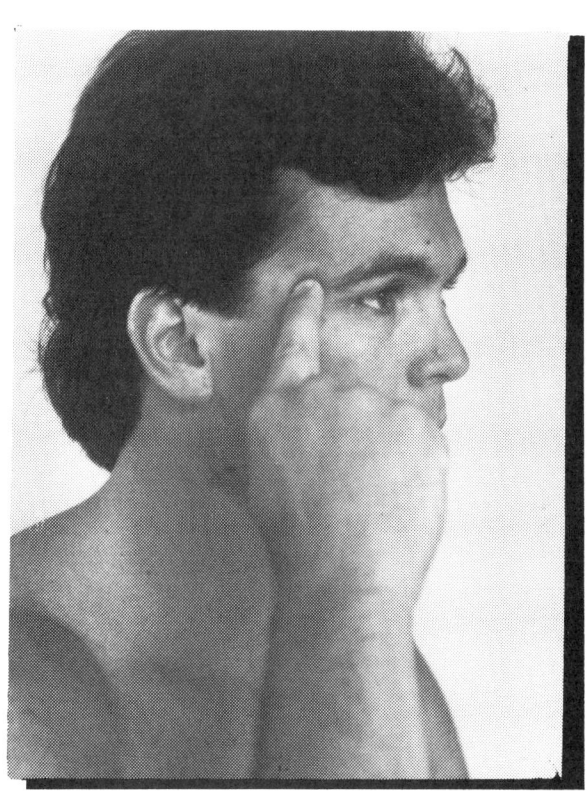

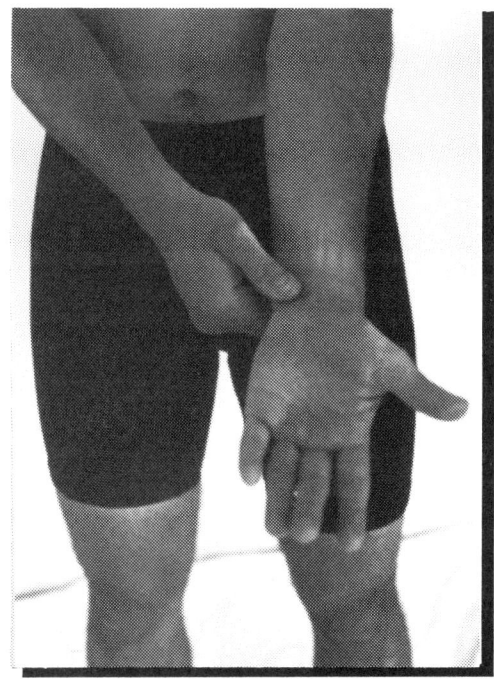

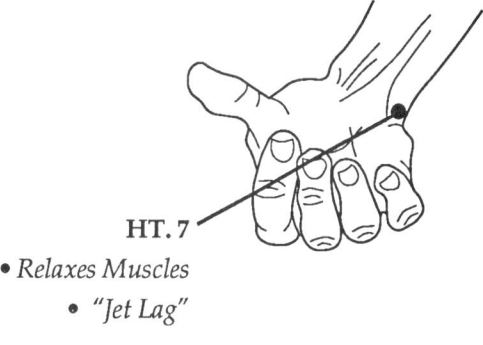

HT. 7
• *Relaxes Muscles*
• *"Jet Lag"*

Illustrations by Judy Smith

ACUPRESSURE FOR INCREASED ENERGY AND PERFORMANCE

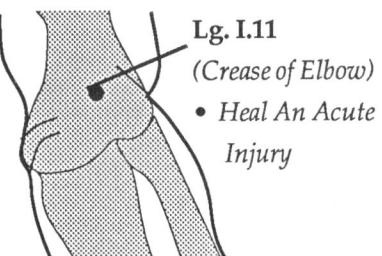

Lg. I.11
(Crease of Elbow)
• *Heal An Acute Injury*

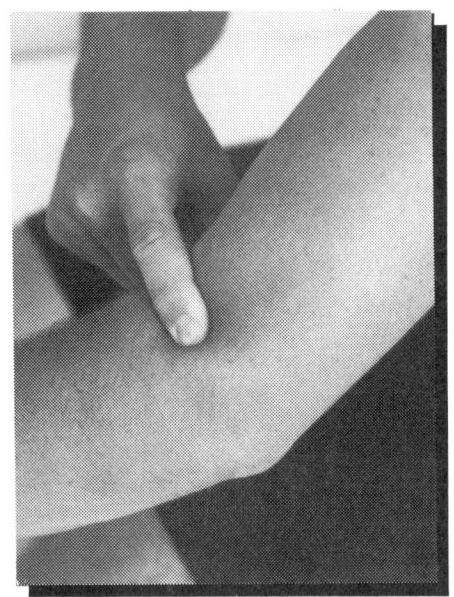

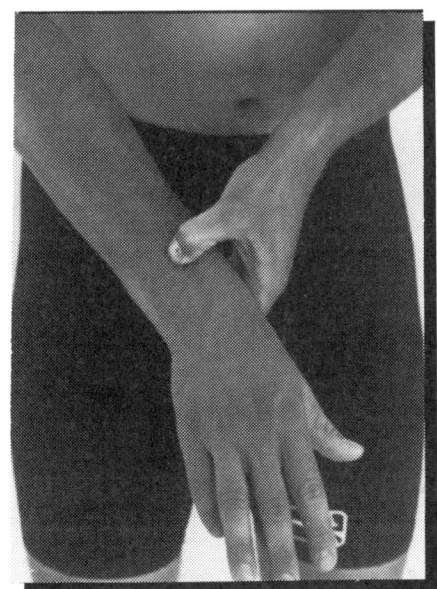

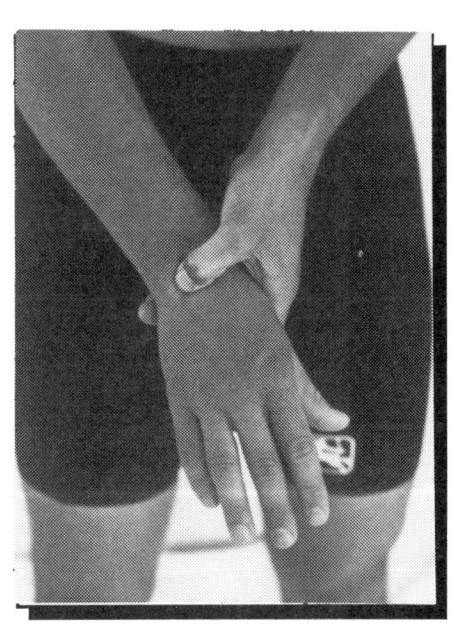

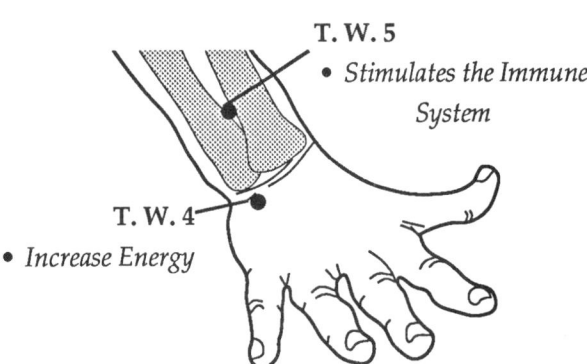

T. W. 5
• *Stimulates the Immune System*

T. W. 4
• *Increase Energy*

Illustrations by Judy Smith

ACUPRESSURE FOR INCREASED ENERGY AND PERFORMANCE

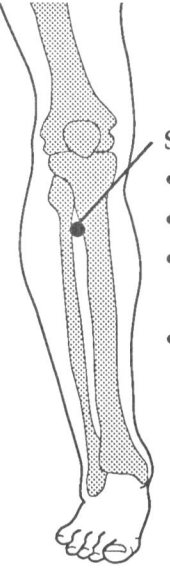

ST. 36
- *Vitality*
- *Heal An Acute Injury*
- *Stimulates the Immune System*
- *Stamina/Balance*

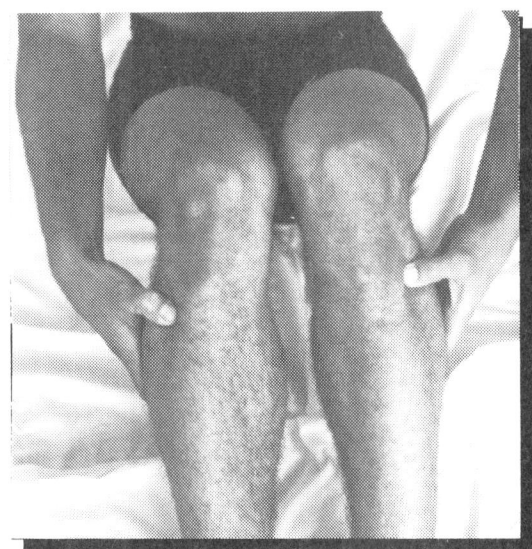

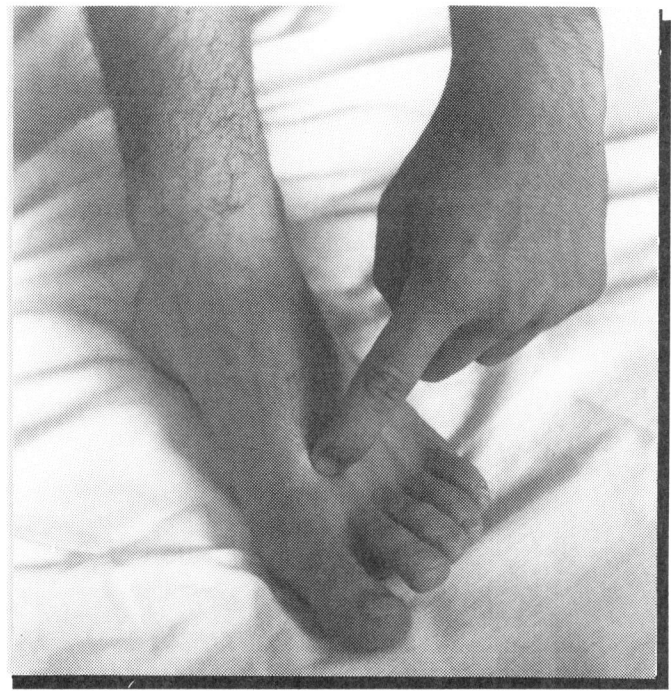

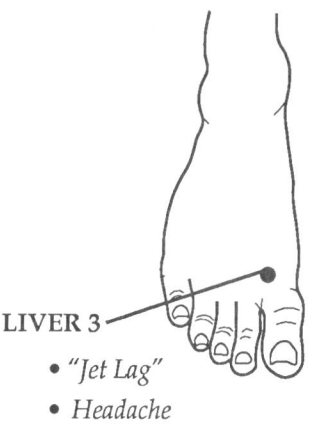

LIVER 3
- *"Jet Lag"*
- *Headache*

Illustrations by Judy Smith

ACUPRESSURE FOR INCREASED ENERGY AND PERFORMANCE

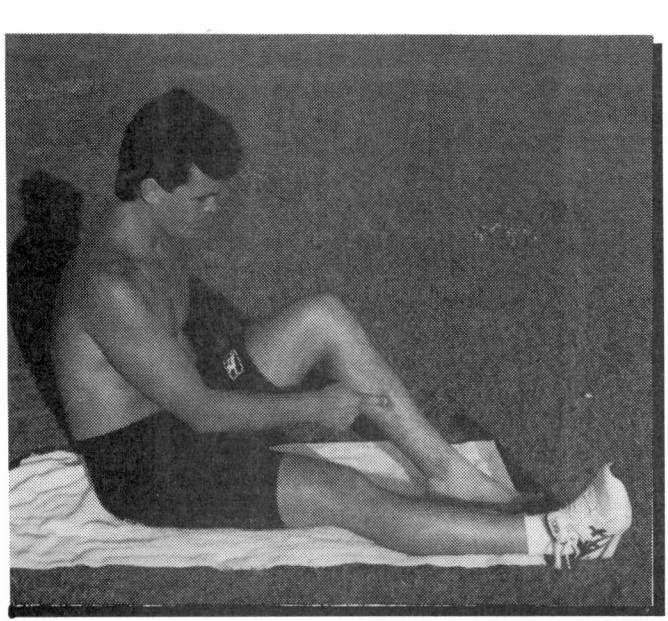

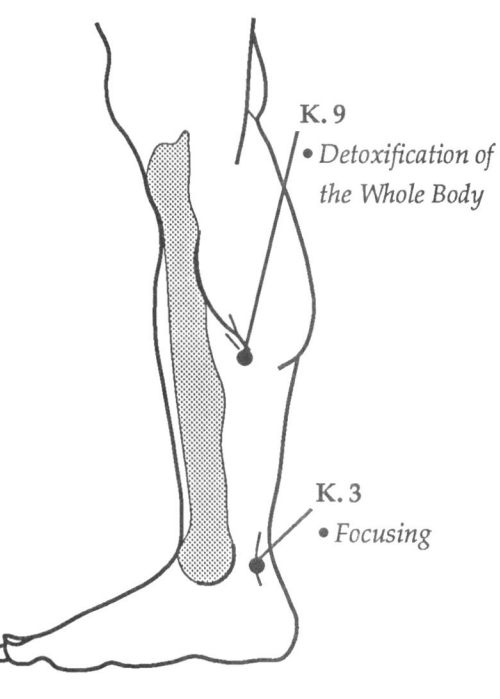

K. 9
• *Detoxification of the Whole Body*

K. 3
• *Focusing*

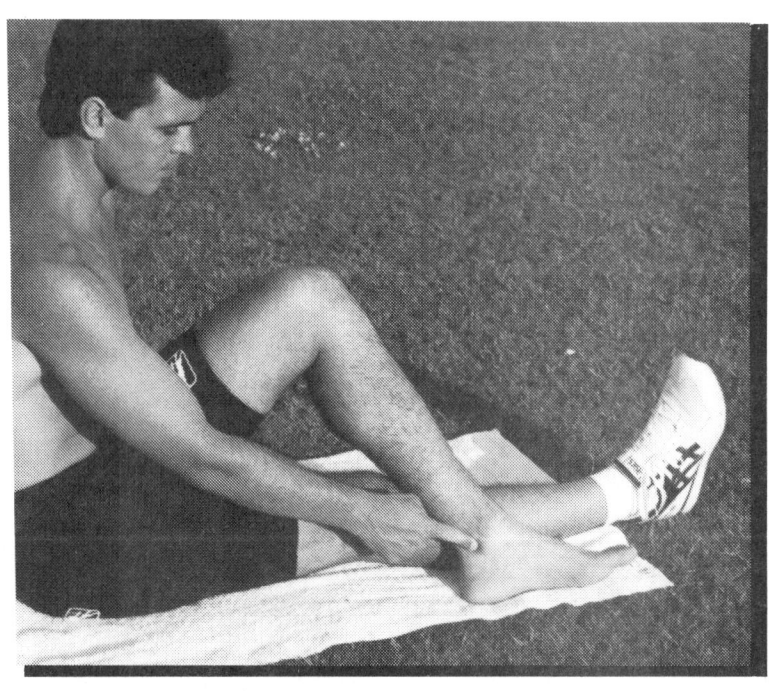

Illustrations by Judy Smith

ACUPRESSURE FOR INCREASED ENERGY AND PERFORMANCE

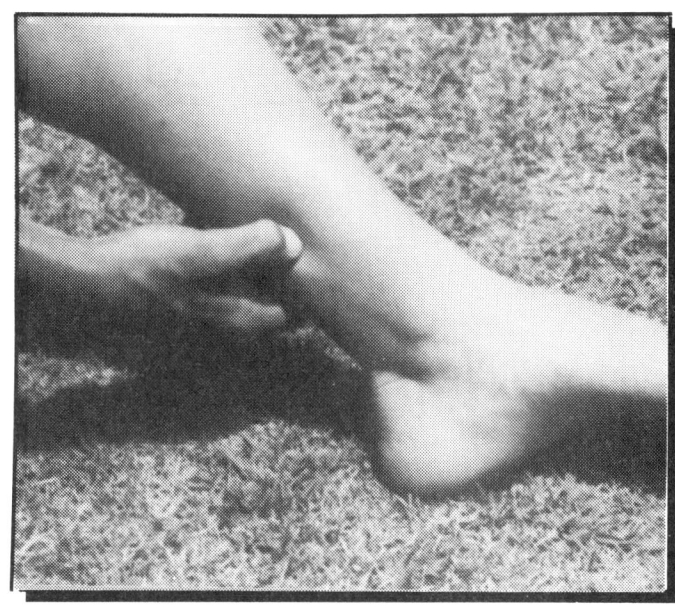

SPL. 6
- *Stimulates the Immune System*

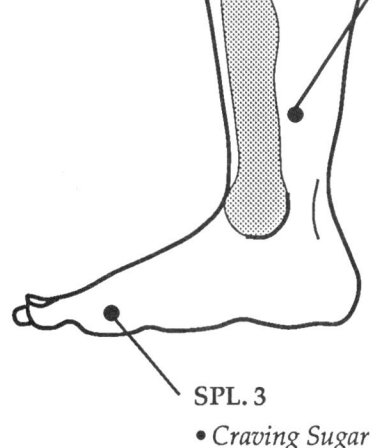

SPL. 3
- *Craving Sugar*

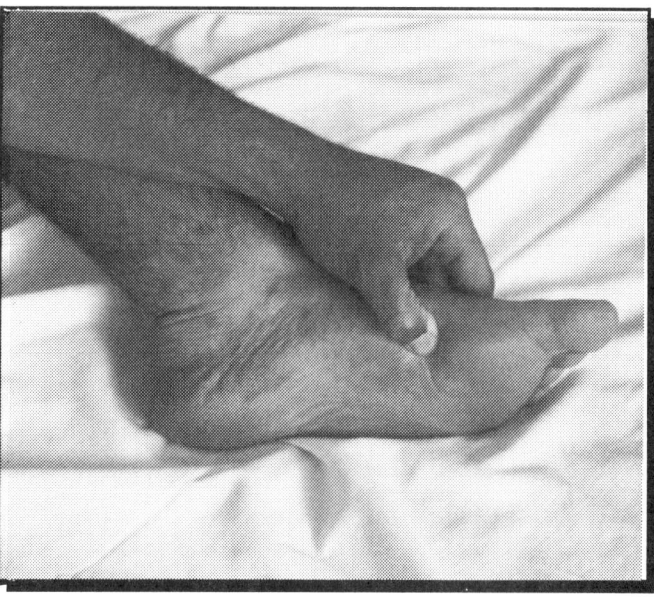

Illustrations by Judy Smith

INFUSE AND CLEANSE

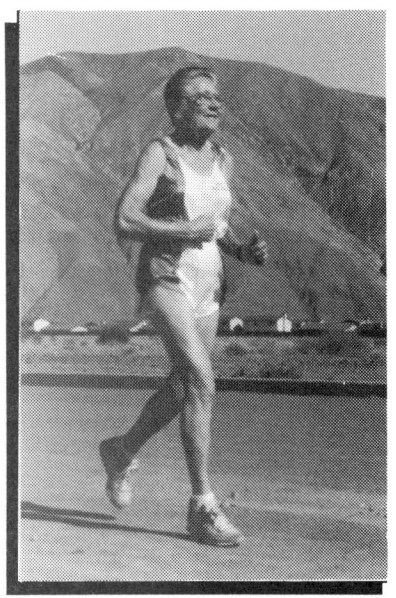

Bess James

Holder of the world record at 5,000 meters at age 75 in a time of 29:19; the American holder at 5,000 meters in a time of 27:25 at age 74; at the 10,000 meter distance, Bess holds the American record for ages 69, 70, 71 and 74 with a best time of 60:01 at age 70.

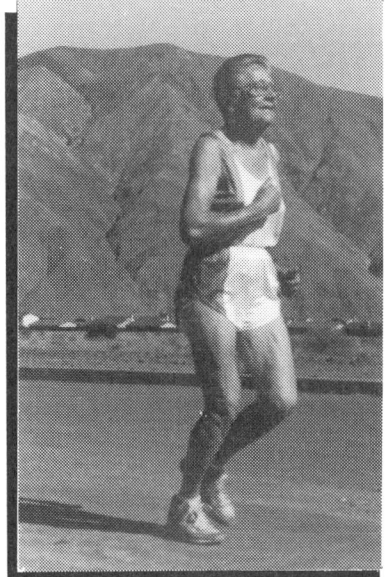

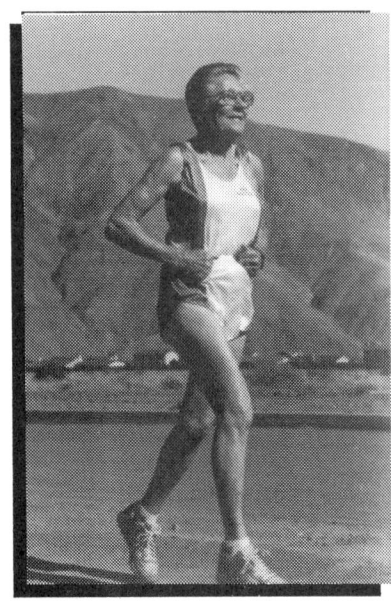

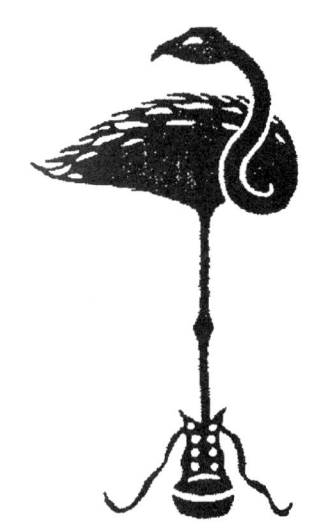

INFUSE & CLEANSE
NEURO -LYMPHATIC REFLEXES (CLEANSE)

Neuro-lymphatic reflex points, known as "the Chapman Reflexes" were first discovered by Frank Chapman, D.O. These reflexes are located mainly along the rib cage, on the abdomen, down the spinal column, and some on the arms and legs.

An active neuro-lymphatic is tender to the touch. Massaging firmly and deeply and providing stimulation for one to five minutes or maybe longer, will usually clear the reflex. However, the precise definition of "clear" will vary from person to person.

George Goodheart, D.C. made the correlation between the neuro-lymphatic points and specific muscles. By firmly rubbing the neuro-lymphatic associated with a particular muscle, one can see dramatic improvement in strength and function.

In my practice, I have found that by showing my athletes the neuro-lymphatics associated with their hardest-worked muscles, they could apply self-massage and keep both the muscle and the reflex clear. This prevents fatigue and eventual spasm from metabolic waste build-up, which shows up in the form of soreness, stiffness and pain.

In competitions, especially endurance races, consistent rubbing of the neuro-lymphatics keeps the muscles fresh and unfatigued, even under extreme stress. As you can imagine, this gives the athlete quite an edge over his competitors by increased endurance, strength and stamina.

INFUSE & CLEANSE
NEURO-VASCULAR REFLEXES (INFUSE)

In the 1930's, Terence Bennett, D.C., discovered points on the head which influence the vascularity (infusion of blood) to the organs and muscles.

Then in the 1960's, George Goodheart D.C. discovered that lightly touching these points improved muscular function. Many of these reflex points affect more then just one muscle; most of them are located on the front of the body and the head, although some can be found on the legs.

By lightly touching a reflex point, then holding it approximately twenty seconds and waiting for a pulsation under the skin, you can improve muscle function and strength by "INFUSING" blood directly into the muscle.

INFUSE AND CLEANSE

INFUSE – INCREASE CIRCULATION

CLEANSE – DRAIN WASTE FROM SORE MUSCLES

Neuro-Vascular points are mainly located on the head. They appear to improve circulation to muscles and organs, increasing their strength. Lightly hold for 30 seconds or longer.

Neuro-Lymphatic points are located in the front and back of the body. The lymphatic system works as a drainage system to "cleanse" waste products from sore muscles. By rubbing these areas deeply 30 seconds to 5 minutes, balance and energy will be restored to the muscle.

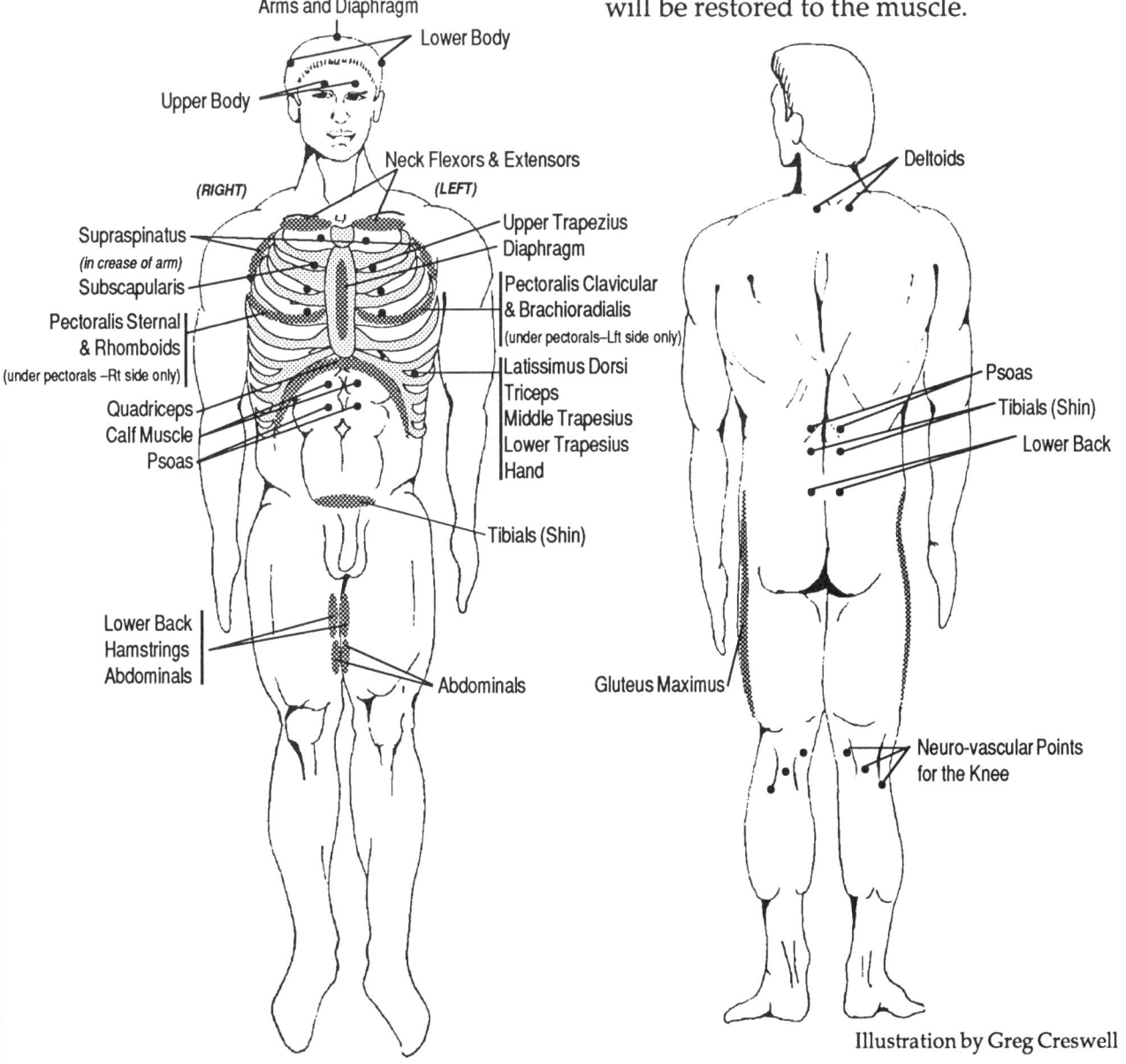

Arms and Diaphragm
Lower Body
Upper Body
Neck Flexors & Extensors
(RIGHT)
(LEFT)
Supraspinatus
(in crease of arm)
Subscapularis
Pectoralis Sternal & Rhomboids
(under pectorals –Rt side only)
Quadriceps
Calf Muscle
Psoas
Upper Trapezius
Diaphragm
Pectoralis Clavicular & Brachioradialis
(under pectorals–Lft side only)
Latissimus Dorsi
Triceps
Middle Trapesius
Lower Trapesius
Hand
Tibials (Shin)
Lower Back
Hamstrings
Abdominals
Abdominals

Deltoids
Psoas
Tibials (Shin)
Lower Back
Gluteus Maximus
Neuro-vascular Points for the Knee

Illustration by Greg Creswell

STRETCHING

"With regard to preparation before, and recovery after a training session or competition, the single most important aid to athletic performance is stretching and flexibility.

Anyone who does not improve and maintain his or her suppleness is not serious about their sport."

Tony Allen-Cooksey
American and
   World Record Holder
   in the Pentathlon, 1981
Decathlete for 10 years

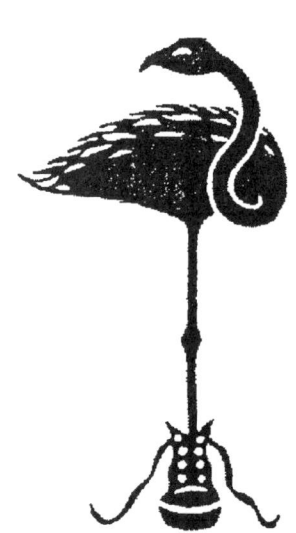

STRETCHING

Up until the twentieth century, almost everyone lived a physically active life. But in today's world, with all its work-saving conveniences, we have two types of people; sedentary and active. People who are sedentary, whether due to illness, old age or just "couch potato-itis," don't use their muscles as much as they could and should. This creates stiffness, soreness and sometimes significant pain. But active people who run, bike, or play tennis also experience soreness and stiffness in their muscles due to overuse. So how do you win?

By stretching daily, before and after a workout, you can increase your body's flexibility and speed your recovery time from soreness and pain while reducing the chance of incurring injury from tight muscles, (Example - too tight hamstrings, shin splints, achilles tendonitis).

Tony Allen-Cooksey, American and world record holder in the Pentathlon (1981) and a decathlete for ten years, says stretching is a must in his training regiment and especially in competition. In training, Tony would warm-up and stretch 30 minutes to 45 minutes prior to training and for competition, 1 hour minimum warm-up and stretching. Stretching can also eliminate overall tension and stress throughout the entire body.

When it is done correctly, stretching feels good. It should never produce moans and groans. When starting out, only go as far as it is comfortable to reach or bend — without straining or bouncing. Stretching incorrectly not only hurts, but can cause serious harm.

So, believe me when I say that stretching does not have to be painful to be effective. I recommend breathing with each stretch as a way of maintaining a fluid rhythm of the body. (If you hold your breath during a stretch, it is much harder to bend or lift). Try it and see! Proper stretching is not stressful and should be incorporated into your daily program of exercise as one of your "Rituals." If you haven't stretched you really aren't ready to start the day, let alone participate in your favorite sport. You are at high risk for an injury to occur, "An accident looking to happen."

STRETCHING

Goals of Stretching

1. To Increase Flexibility
2. To Reduce Stress and Tension in the Muscles
3. To Reduce the Chance of Injuries

Instructions

1. Never Force a Stretch and Never BOUNCE
2. Focus on your breathing as a way to release tension throughout the body.
3. Work towards the 30 - 60 second goal even if you can't do anymore than 10 seconds a day.

HOW TO STRETCH

1.   Never go out "cold" when you engage in any form of sport or exercise.

2.   Warm-up for a good 10-15 minutes, in order to get your blood fully circulating (Example - jog a mile, cycle for 15 minutes, 100 light jumping jacks). You'll find that it is easier to stretch "warm" than "cold".

3.   Stretch for 15-20 minutes, then continue on with your exercise routine.

4.   After exercise, "warm-down" until your heart rate is below 100. You never want to just stop exercising. You want the heart to slow down gradually. This normalizes heart rate and circulation throughout the body.

5.   Now stretch for 20-30 minutes, relaxing and breathing into each stretch. This way you won't become stiff or sore the next day.

Properly combined, a routine of exercise and stretching will relieve stress and improve circulation and lymphatic flow. It will also flush out toxins which make you feel sluggish and easily fatigued. No matter what time of day you choose to exercise or engage in sports, it's wise to take the time for a brief morning workout just to get your blood moving and your "battery charged". As little as 15 minutes will provide a quick but crucial warm-up to get your day off to the right start. (That doesn't mean, however, that you should "hit the floor running.") Warm-up slowly and sensibly, paying attention, as always, to your body's signals.

You'll find that life will be more enjoyable, for you will feel better while you create a foundation on which to build a healthy and optimally fit body.

EXTRA TIP: Remember to drink plenty of water during exercise to prevent dehydration.

EXTRA TIP: To help get rid of the soreness, take a hot epsom salts bath (2 cups in a hot bath) after a workout or sporting event. Epsom salts helps to pull poisons and toxins from the muscles. Soak for 15 minutes. *Do not take a hot bath prior to a sporting event.* It will make you sluggish for the event.

STRETCHES
FULL BODY MUSCULATURE

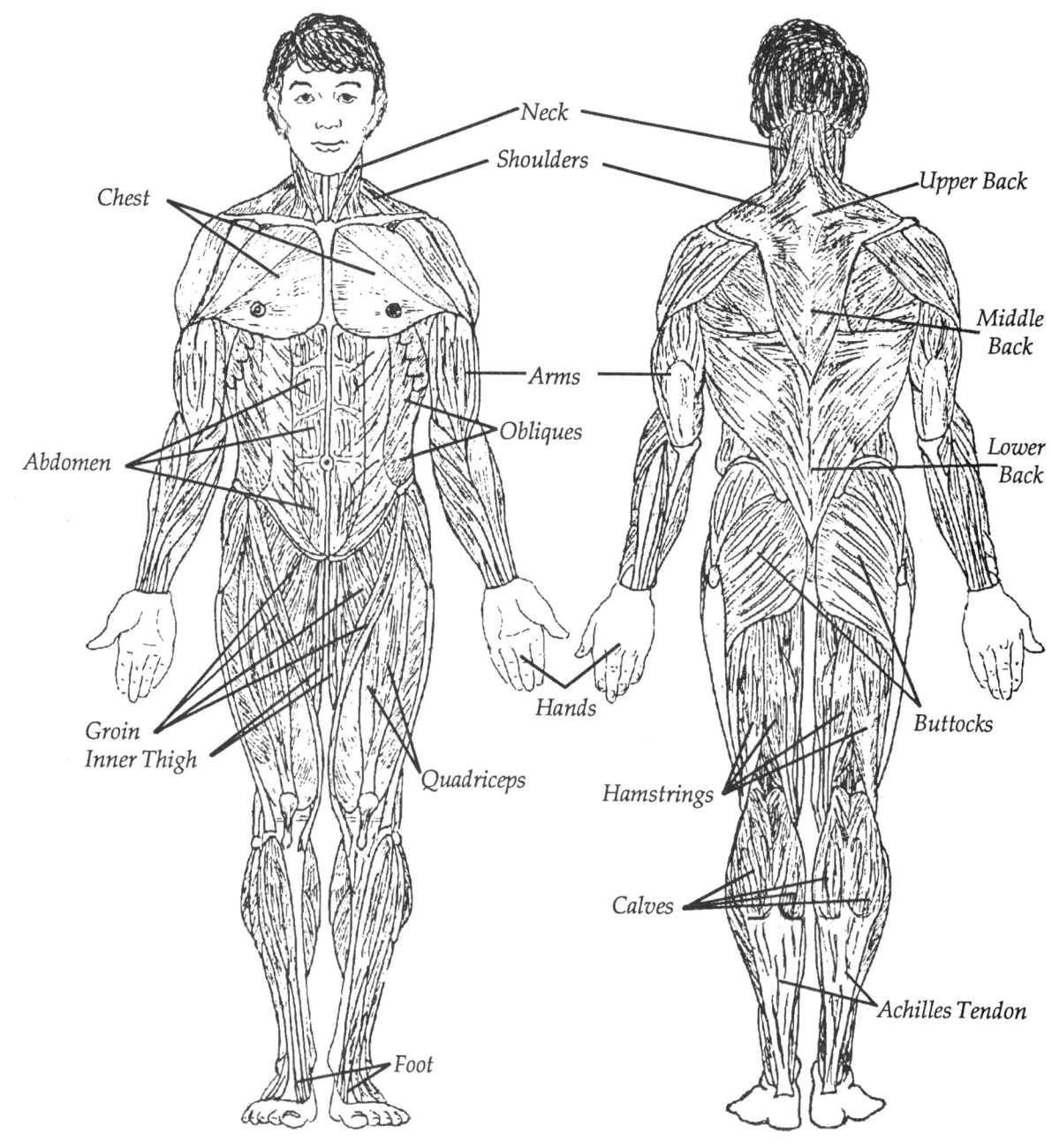

Neck

Shoulders

Chest

Upper Back

Middle Back

Arms

Obliques

Lower Back

Abdomen

Hands

Groin
Inner Thigh

Buttocks

Quadriceps

Hamstrings

Calves

Achilles Tendon

Foot

STRETCHES

1. KNEE TO CHEST

Position: Lie on back, bring **right** leg to chest while **left** leg is bent. This reduces stress on the low-back. Hold this position 30-60 seconds. Switch legs and repeat stretch.

Breathing: **Inhale** as you raise leg and **exhale** as it reaches the chest. Continue to breathe diaphragmatically for 30-60 seconds.

Purpose: To release tension in the low-back, buttock muscles, and quadriceps (upper thigh muscles).

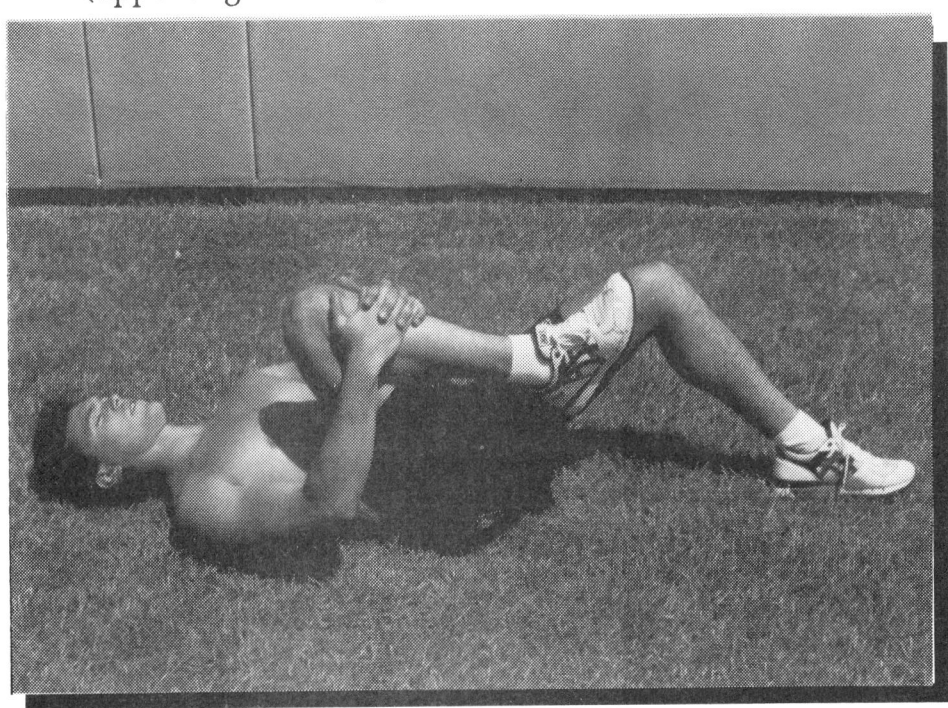

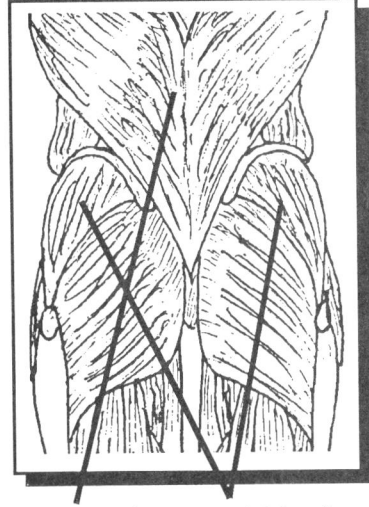

Lower Back & Buttock Muscles

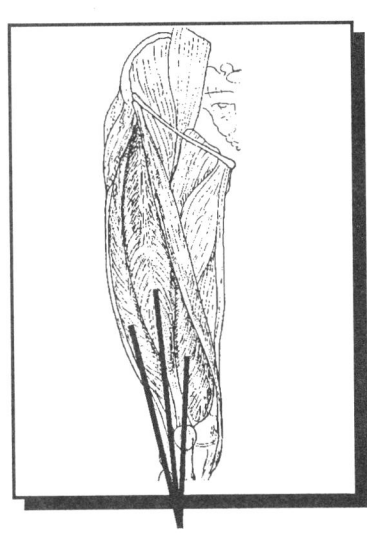

Quadriceps
(Upper Thigh Muscles)

STRETCHES

2. KNEES TO CHEST

Position: Lie on back. Bring **both** knees to the chest.

Breathing: **Inhale** as you raise both legs, (knees).**Exhale** as upper legs (knees) reach chest. Continue to diaphragmatically breathe for 30-60 seconds.

As you breathe, relax the jaw, shoulders, back and legs.

Purpose: To release tension in the low-back,buttock and quadricep muscles.

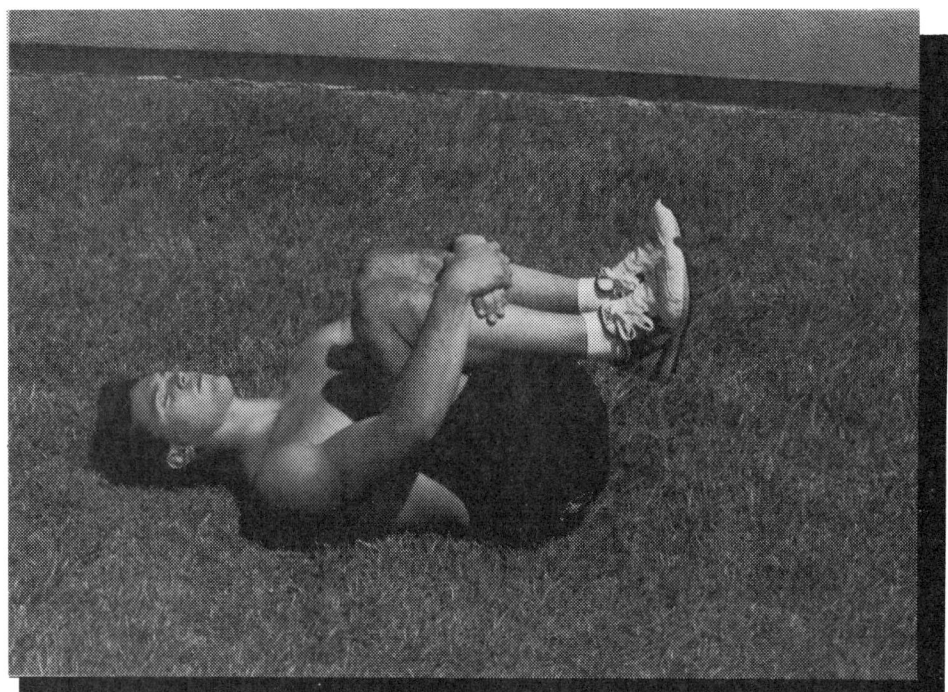

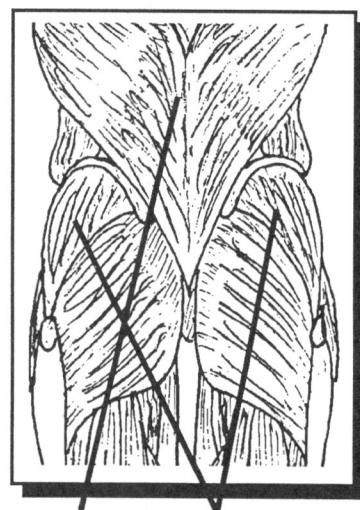

Lower Back & Buttock Muscles

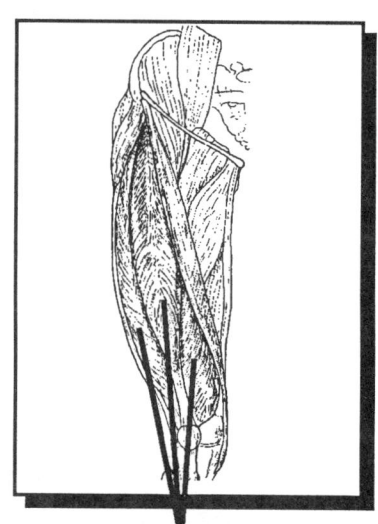

Quadriceps
(Upper Thigh Muscles)

STRETCHES
3. HEEL TO SKY

Position: Lie on back: Bring **right** leg to chest, place hands *behind* knee, keeping knee in same place, extend lower leg, then flex foot, toes toward head, heel toward sky.

Breathing: **Inhale** as you raise leg to chest. **Exhale**. **Inhale** as you extend lower leg. **Exhale. Inhale** as you flex foot, toes toward head, heel to sky. **Exhale.** Hold stretch and continue to diaphragmatically breathe 30-60 seconds.

Purpose: To release tension and stretch the low-back, buttock muscles, hamstrings, calves, and achilles tendon.

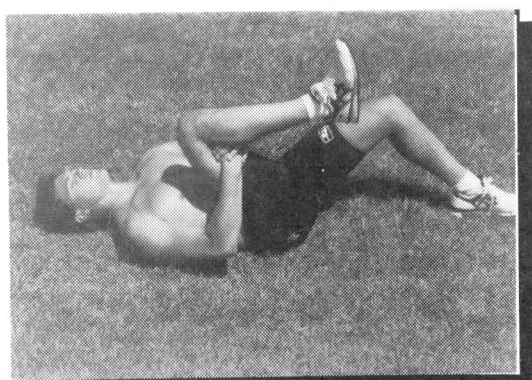

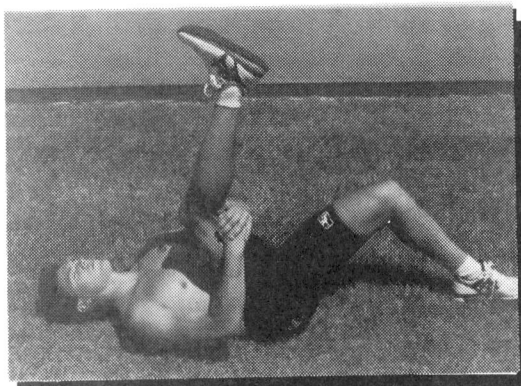

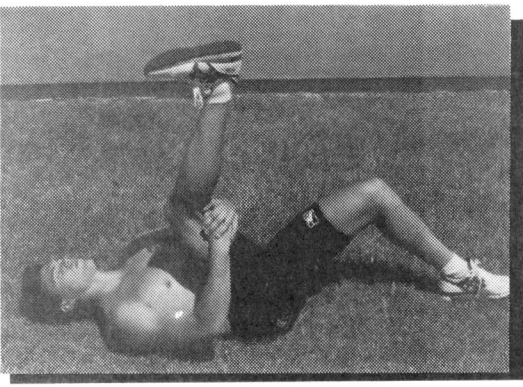

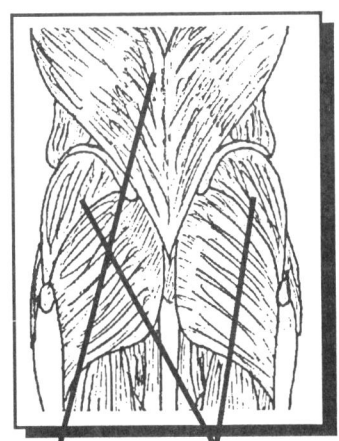

Lower Back & Buttock Muscles

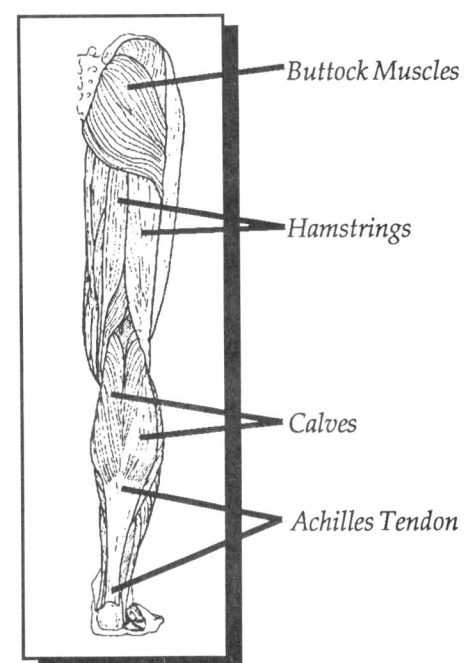

Buttock Muscles

Hamstrings

Calves

Achilles Tendon

STRETCHES

4. RESPIRATORY SPINAL EXTENSION (Spinal Twist)

Position: Lie on back, arms extended to side, bend **right** leg to 90 degrees, flex foot slowly, rotate **right** knee towards floor. Hold position 30-60 seconds.

Breathing: **Inhale** as you bend leg to 90 degrees. **Exhale** as you rotate knee to floor. Continue to diaphragmatically breathe and "let your body go".

Relax your jaw, shoulders, back, and hips.

Purpose: To release tension in the spinal muscles, chest, shoulders, buttock muscles, abdominals and obliques (muscles on the side of the body.)

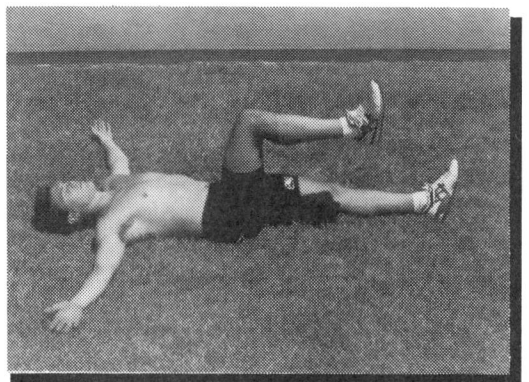 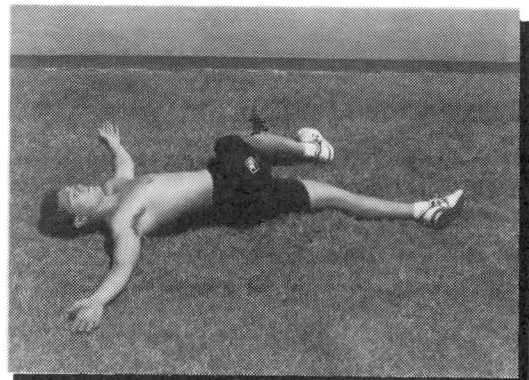

Shoulders

Chest

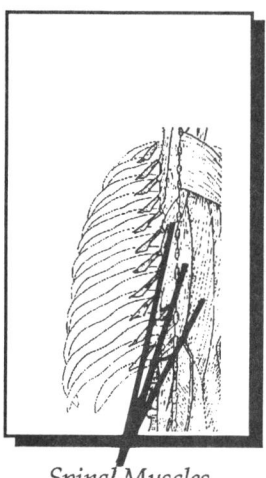 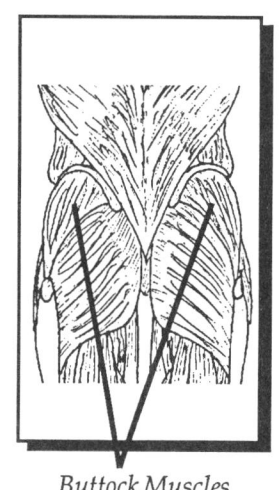 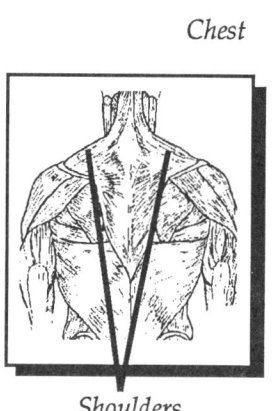 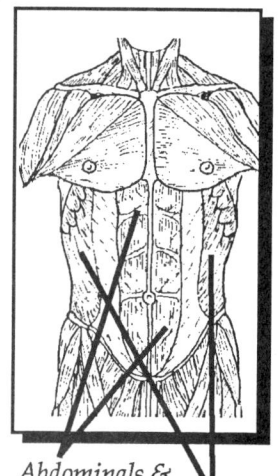

Spinal Muscles   *Buttock Muscles*   *Shoulders*   *Abdominals & Obliques*

STRETCHES
5. SIT AND RELAX

Position: Sitting, legs extended, knees unlocked, arms resting on floor. Lean slightly forward, slowly let head drop.

Relax jaw, neck, and shoulders. "Let your lips hang loose."

Breathe: **Inhale** and **exhale** as you lean forward. Continue to diaphragmatically breathe as you relax. Hold stretch 30-60 seconds.

Purpose: To release tension in the upper, middle, and low back, hamstrings, buttock muscles, shoulders, arms, neck, jaw and face.

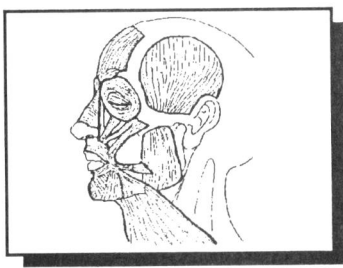

Neck, Jaw & Face Muscles

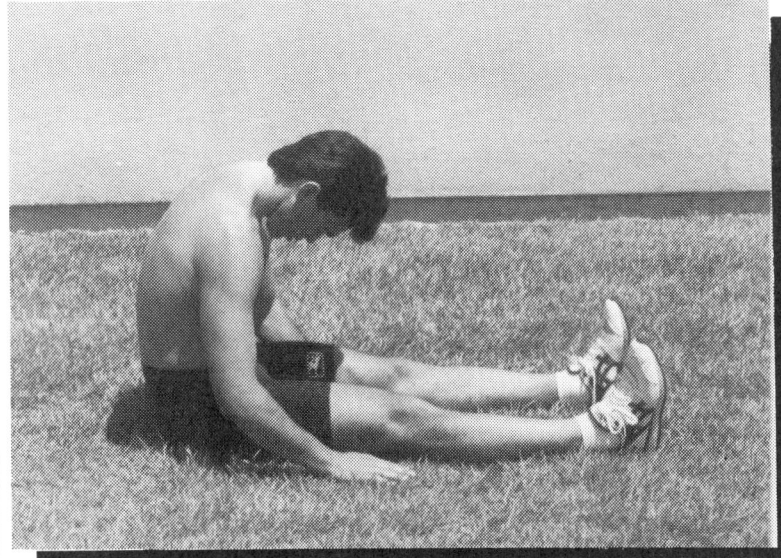

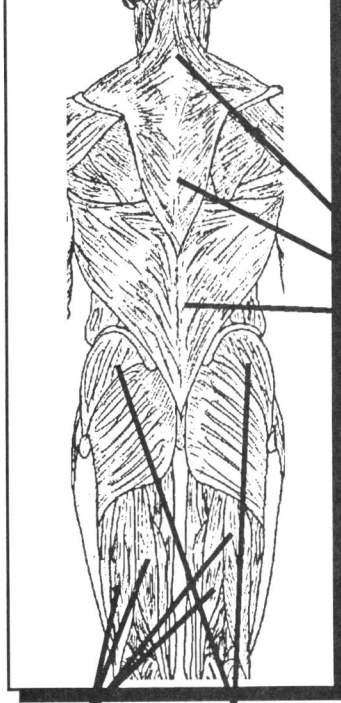

Upper Back
Middle Back
Low Back

Hamstrings & Buttock Muscles

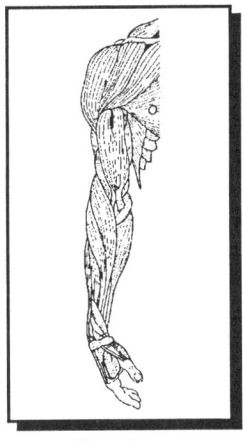

(front)

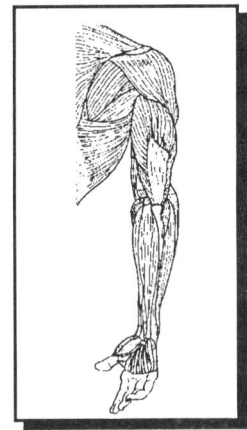

(back)

SHOULDERS & ARMS

STRETCHES

6. SADDLESTRETCH

Position: Sitting, straddle legs apart, arms in front, walk hands forward.

Breathing: **Inhale, exhale** as you lean forward. Continue to breathe as you relax. Hold position 30-60 seconds.

Purpose: To release tension in the upper, middle, and lowback, hamstrings, buttock muscles, inner thigh, groin, shoulders, and arms.

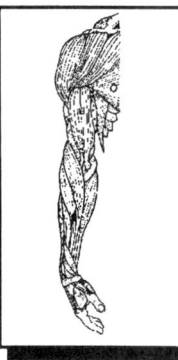

(front)

SHOULDERS & ARMS

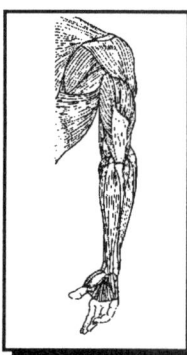

(back)

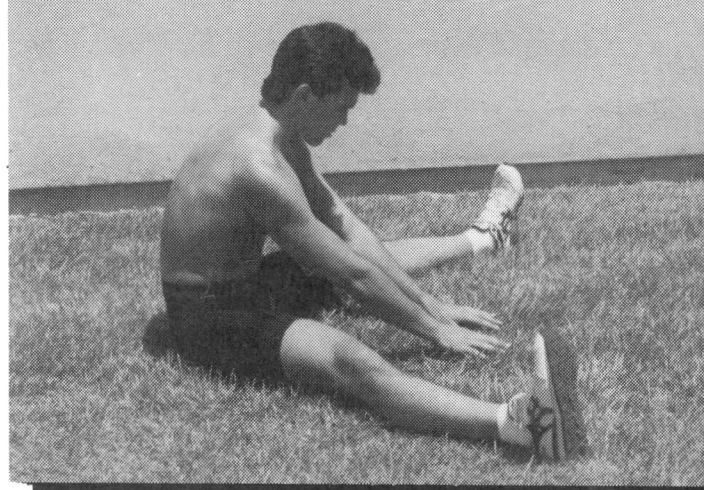

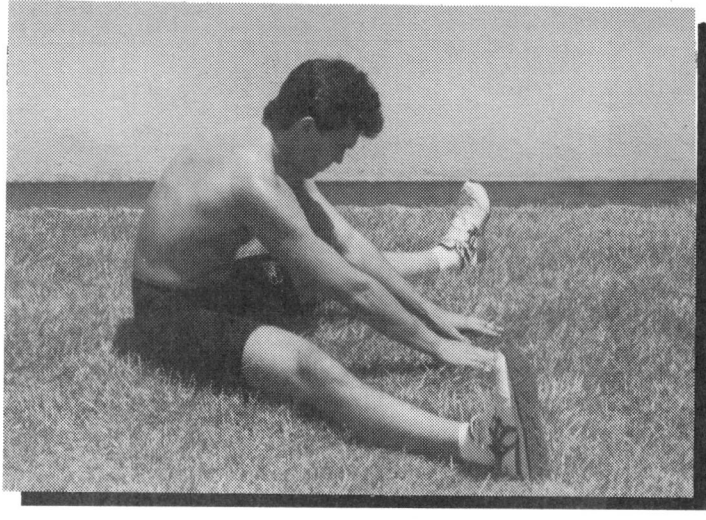

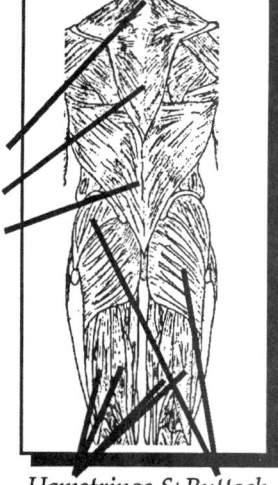

Upper Back

Middle Back

Low Back

Hamstrings & Buttock Muscles

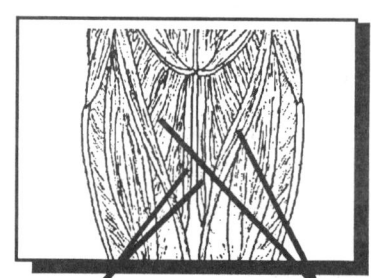

Inner Thigh   *Groin*

STRETCHES
7. QUADRICEP STRETCH

Position: Sitting on heels, sit erect. Hands resting on thighs, head leaning forward, and relaxed. Hold position 30-60 seconds. Relax the back, shoulders, arms, neck, jaw and face.

Breathing: **Inhale** diaphragmatically and **exhale** as you relax each muscle group. Focus.

Purpose: To release tension and stretch quadriceps, lower leg muscles, foot muscles.

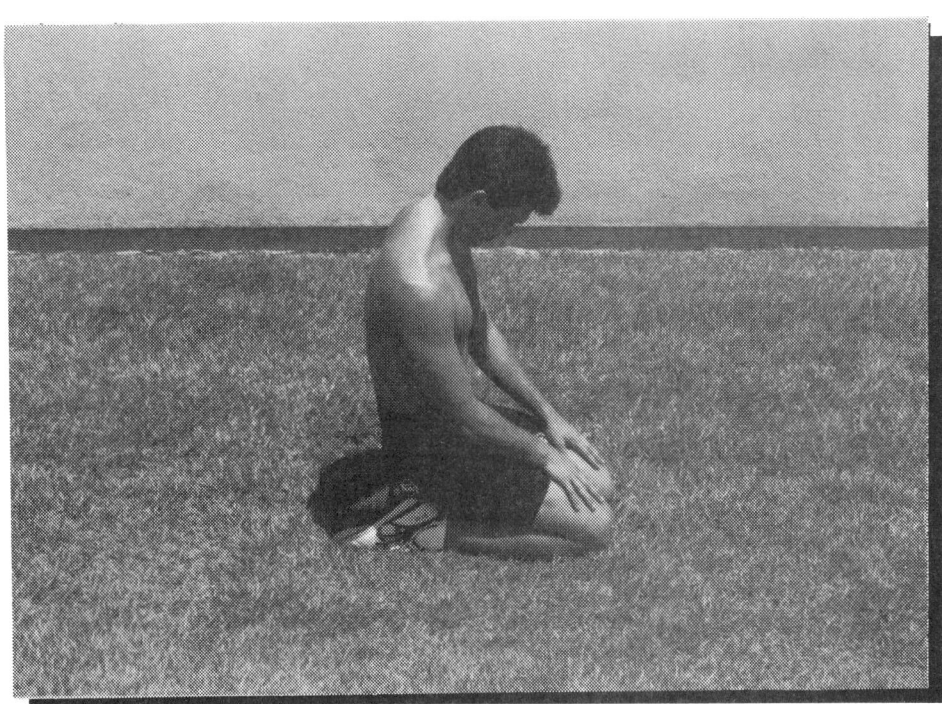

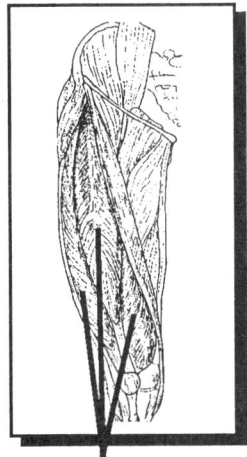

Quadriceps

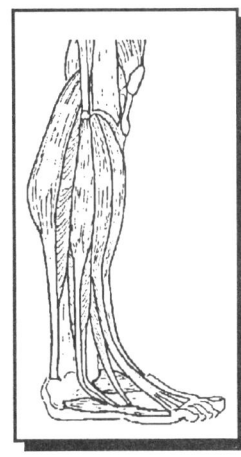

Lower Leg Muscles

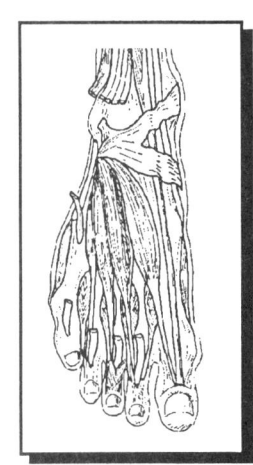

Foot Muscles

STRETCHES

8. HUG YOURSELF

Position: Sitting, standing, or kneeling, wrap your arms around at just below shoulder level. Walk your fingers toward center of back. Hold position 30-60 seconds.

Breathing: **Inhale** diaphragmatically and **exhale** slowly.

Purpose: To release tension in the upper back, shoulders.

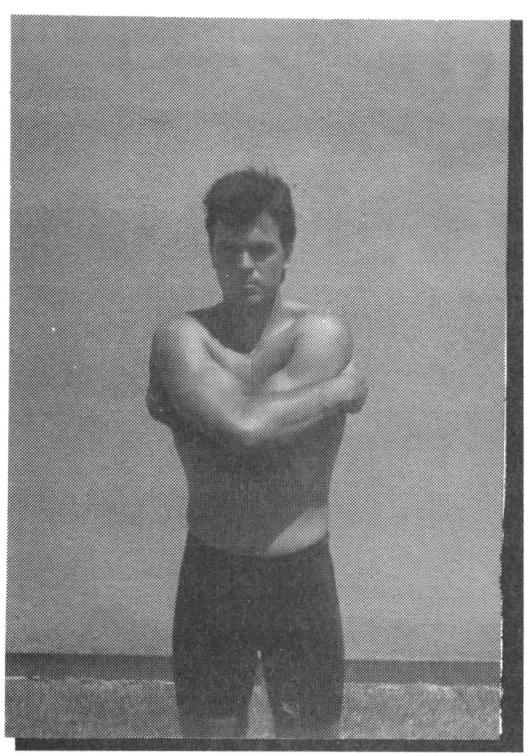
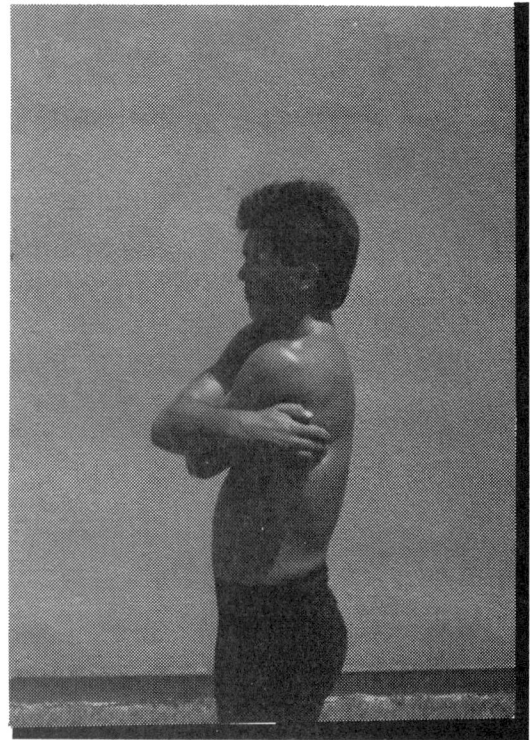

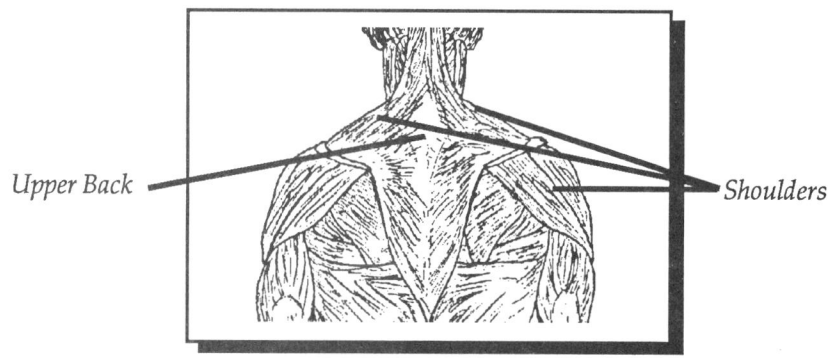

Upper Back   *Shoulders*

STRETCHES
9. REAR ARM EXTENSION

Position: Kneeling, sitting, or standing, arms behind you, clasp hands and lift arms upward. Hold position 30-60 seconds.

Relax the back, shoulders, neck, jaw and face.

Breathing: **Inhale** diaphragmatically. As you **exhale** lift your arms upward.

Purpose: To release tension in the chest muscles, shoulder muscles, arms.

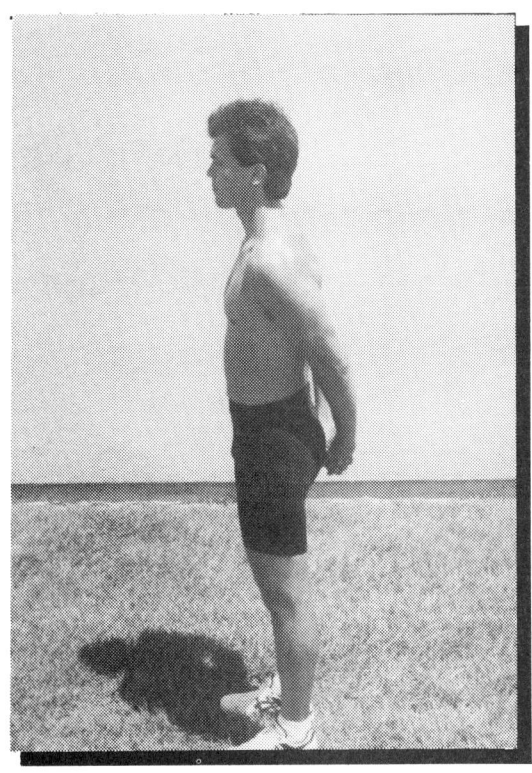 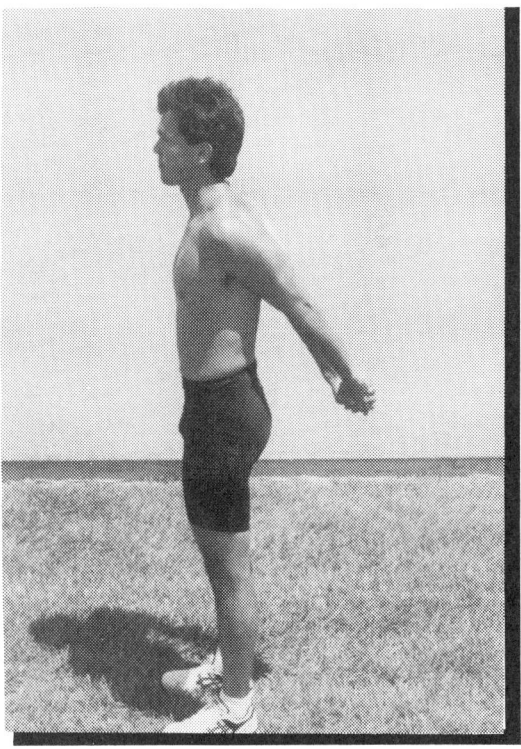

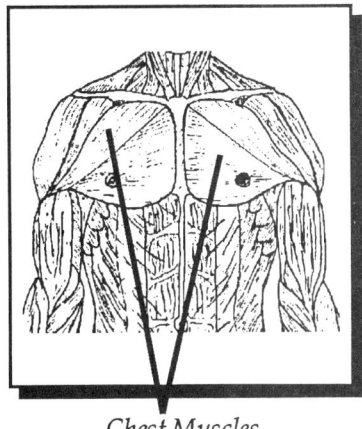

Chest Muscles

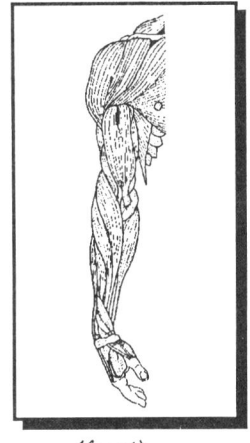

(front)

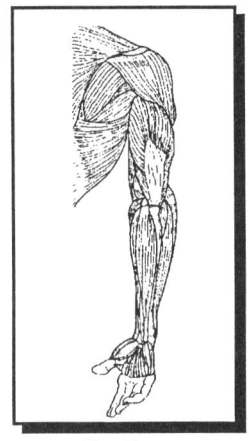

(back)

SHOULDERS & ARMS

STRETCHES

10. SIDE BEND

Position: Standing, raise arms to sky, interlock fingers, keep hips centered. Slowly lean to side, Hold position 30-60 seconds. Now lean to opposite side. Hold position 30-60 seconds.

Relax the back, shoulders, arms, neck, jaw and face.

Breathing: **Inhale. Exhale** as you lean to the side. Continue to breathe as you hold position. **Inhale** up and **exhale** as you lean to the side. Hold Position 30-60 seconds.

Purpose: To release tension in the side muscles, low-back, arms, hands and fingers.

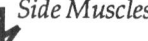
Side Muscles

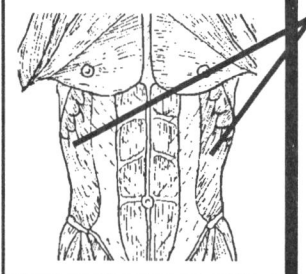

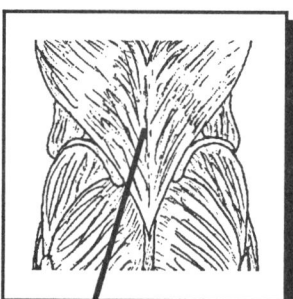
Low-back Muscles

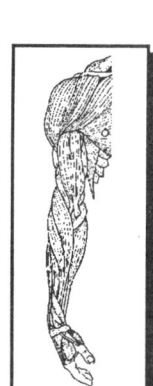
Arms

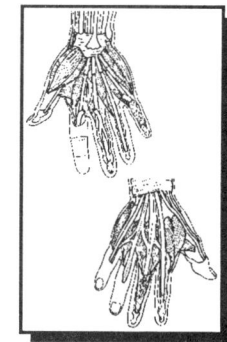
Hands & Fingers

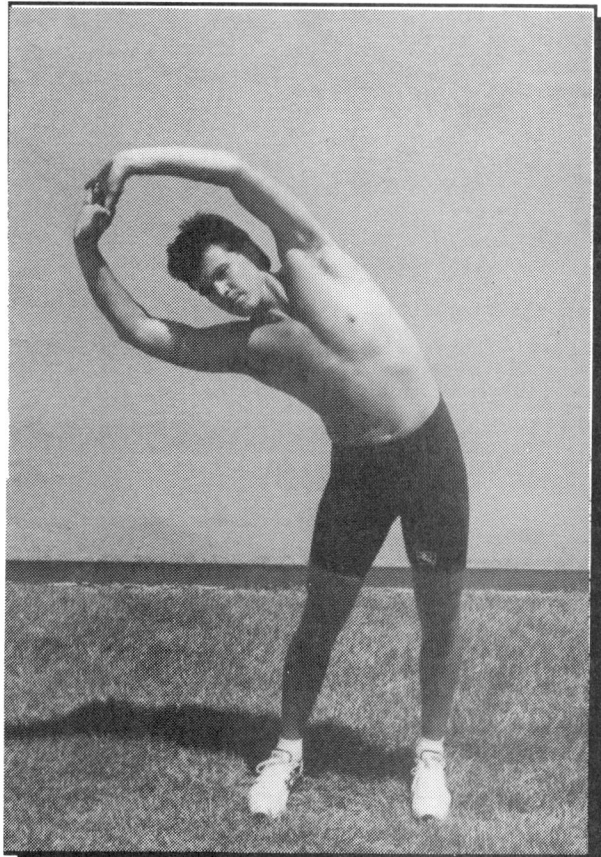

STRETCHES
11. TRUNK TWIST

Position: Standing, hands on hips, feet shoulder width apart, knees slightly bent, twist to the **right**. Hold position 30-60 seconds. Return to center. Slowly twist to the **left**. Hold position 30-60 seconds.

Breathing: **Inhale** in the center position. **Exhale** as you twist.

Purpose: To release tension in the side muscles, abdominals, back, and buttock muscles.

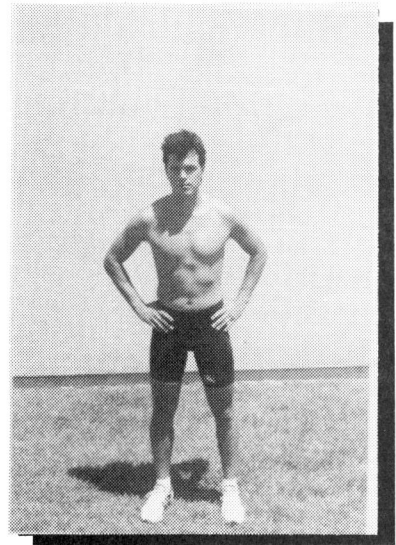

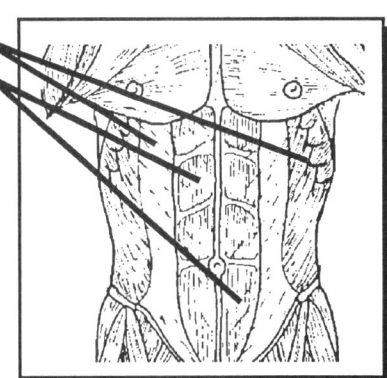

Side Muscles & Abdominals

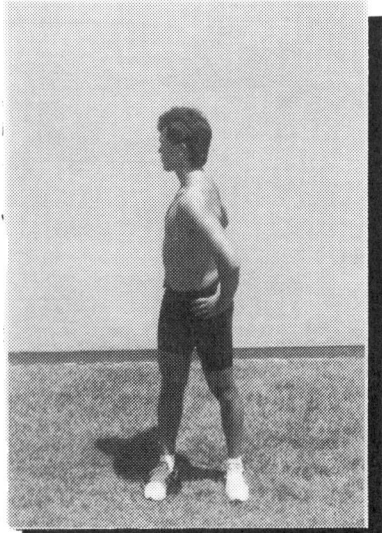

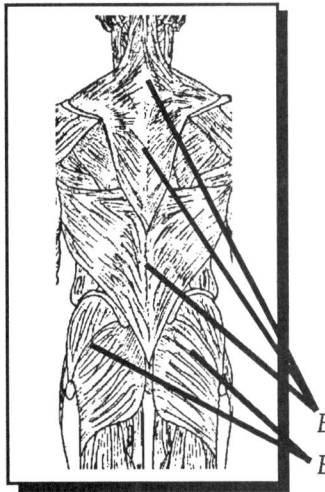

Back Muscles & Buttock Muscles

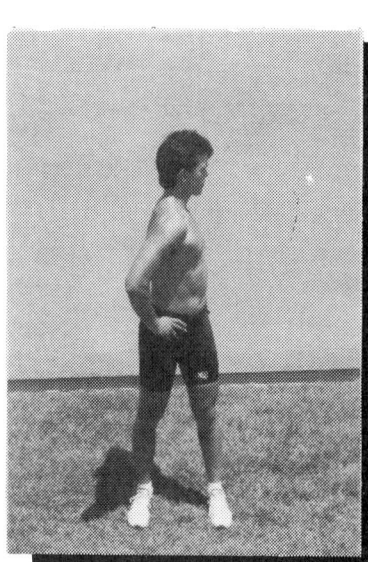

STRETCHES

12. GOOD MORNING

Position: Standing with feet shoulder width apart, knees slightly bent, place hands on hips. Maintain a natural curve of the back: **Slowly** lean forward to 45 degrees. **Allow knees to bend**. Repeat 10 times. Slowly return to standing position and straighten legs.

DO NOT BEND OVER WITH LOCKED KNEES.

MAINTAIN LOW BACK CURVATURE.

Breathing: **Inhale. Exhale** down. **Inhale** up.

Purpose: To release tension and strengthen the low-back, buttock muscles and hamstrings.

THIS MAKES YOU USE YOUR DIAPHRAGM MUSCLE.

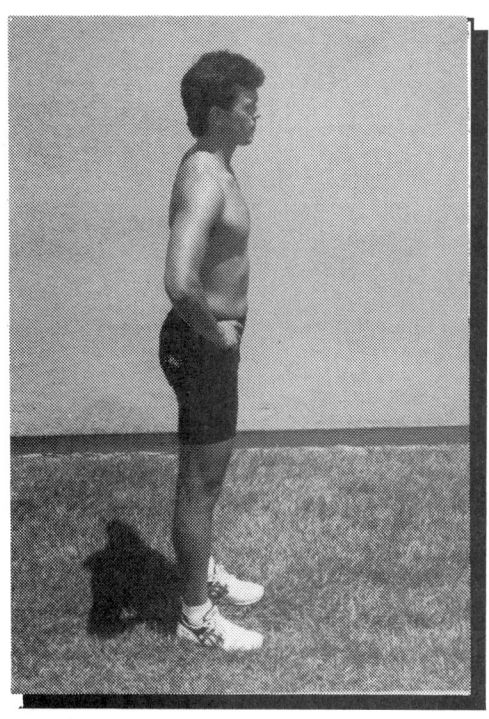
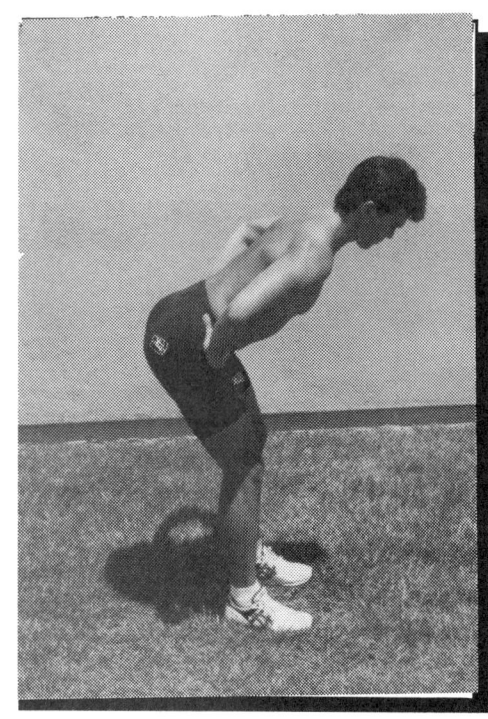

Lower Back &
Buttock Muscles

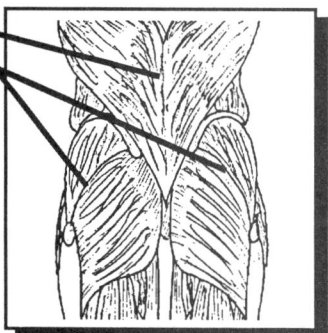

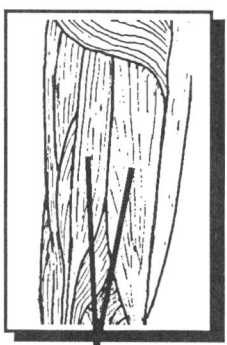

Hamstrings

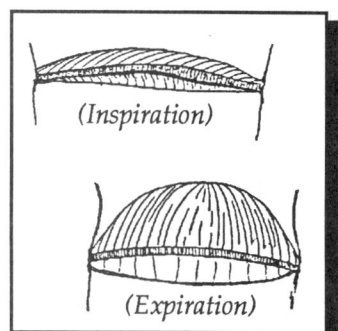

Diaphragm

(Inspiration)

(Expiration)

FOOT PAD RELEASE

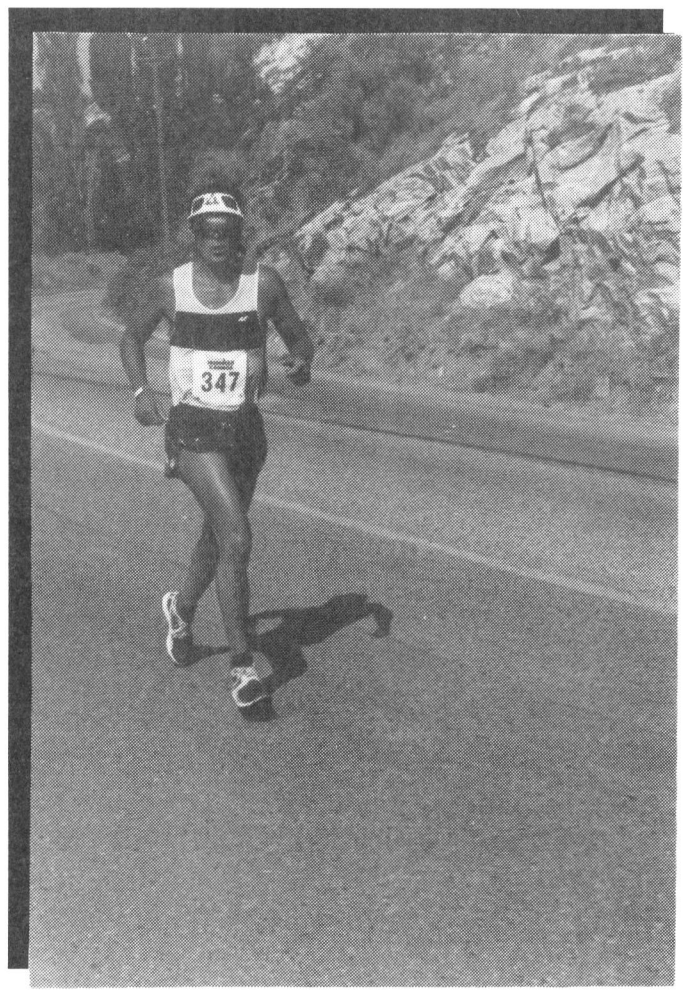

David Hemingway

For the athlete, foot stability is essential for maintaining proper alignment of the whole body.

FOOT PAD RELEASE

For stability and balance, our feet need to be firmly planted on the ground. As obvious as this sounds, it is not quite as simple as you think.

Our feet become unstable for a number of reasons. High heels, overly tight or worn down shoes, and shoes with inadequate arch support can all distort the foot's natural form, causing the tendons and connective tissue to gradually become tight and drawn up.

When three pads on the bottom of the foot (ball, side, and heel) are no longer fully or evenly touching the ground, instability results. Unbalanced feet can lead to a misalignment of your entire body, creating muscle tension. This tension can be the cause of leg pain, lower back pain, neck and shoulder discomfort and headaches.

For the athlete, foot stability is essential for maintaining proper alignment of the whole body.

In any sport you participate in, foot stability will determine how you run, jump, bike, swim, or even when you go hiking.

By spreading and massaging the muscles and tendons on the bottom of the foot, you create a more stable and solid foundation in which to walk. Thus avoiding eventual knee, hip and low-back problems.

By releasing these three foot pads (ball, side, and heel), they once again come in full contact with the ground, restoring stability and balance throughout the body.

FOOT PAD RELEASE

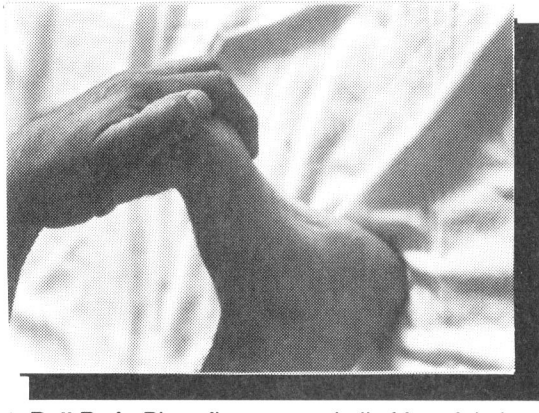

1. Ball Pad • Place fingers over ball of foot. Inhale. Exhale and drag fingers up over ball and through toes while extending foot. (3 reps)

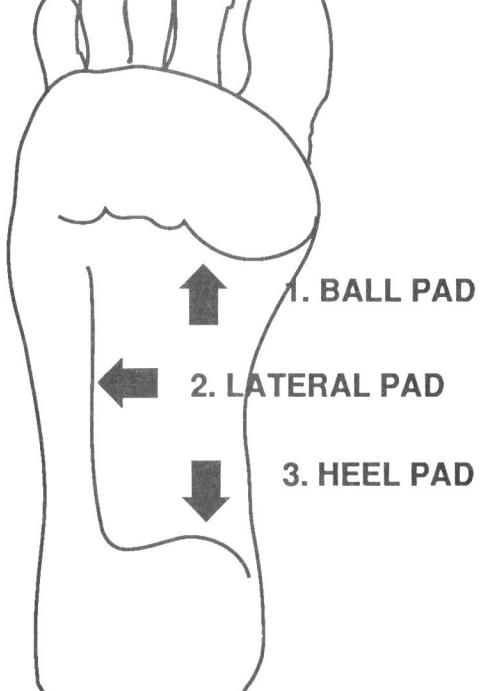

1. BALL PAD

2. LATERAL PAD

3. HEEL PAD

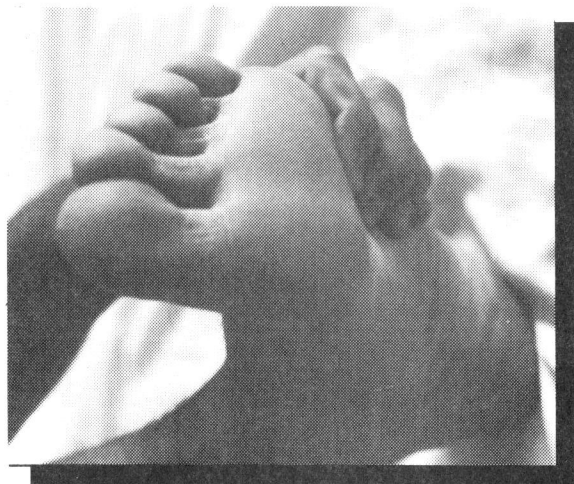

2. Lateral Pad • Place fingers along bottom surface of foot in the soft tissue. Inhale. Exhale and drag fingers toward the outside of foot while rotating foot inward. (3 reps)

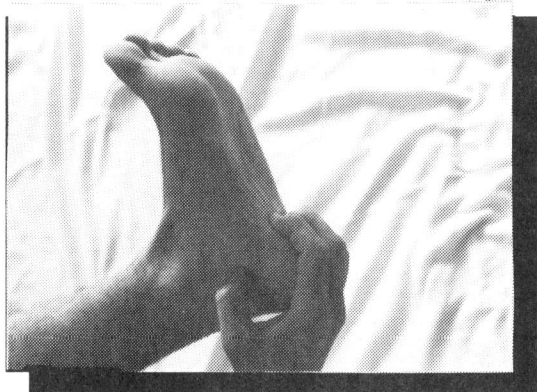

3. Heel Pad • Place fingers in the soft tissue area in front of heel. Inhale. Exhale and drag fingers over heel surface while flexing foot. (3 reps)

Illustration by Greg Creswell

VISUALIZATION

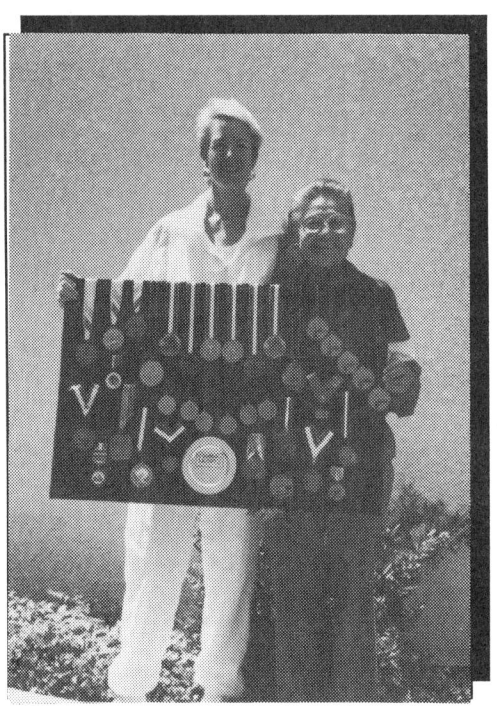

Bess James and myself

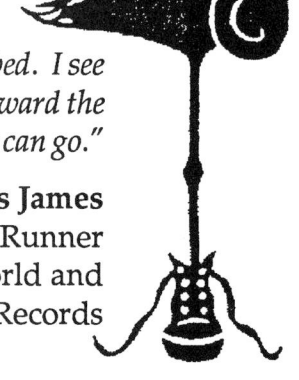

"I find a quiet place away from anyone I know, so I won't be disturbed. I see myself doing the actual race, taking off as fast as possible, sprinting toward the finish line, moving my arms and legs in perfect form and as fast as they can go."

— Bess James
Masters Runner
Holder of World and
American Records

VISUALIZATION

Whether you are an athlete, a business person, or a student, **mental training prepares you for what is to come** — in a race, a meeting or in the classroom. Mental training is just as important as physical training, for the mind and body work together and strongly impact on one another. As you know, the mind is a very powerful computer. As athletes if we program our brains with the proper techniques, we can be well prepared when we go into an event. If we have properly previsioned our moves and responses, when it comes time for the actual competition, our body will be on auto-pilot, focused and running according to our selected "tape".

HOW TO VISUALIZE

Visualization should be done in quiet and peaceful surroundings where you won't be disturbed. Get into a comfortable position (either sitting or lying down) then loosen your clothing and use diaphragmatic breathing to relax your body.

1. Start by visualizing your event
    (running a race, skiing, cycling, swimming, etc.)

2. Imagine your body in position, going through all the motions necessary for your sport. Example: A sprinter in the starting blocks sets himself, rises, the gun goes off and he sprints forward, one foot in front of the other, arms pumping hard ' - to give him the momentum to go even faster — until he crosses the finish line.

    This mental "tape" is a reconstructing of the actual event created by visualizing proper techniques, foot placement, hand-arm placement and body movement. It is a method of instilling the proper images into your "Computer-Brain." It is a first person scenario in which you write, direct and star.

3. Now, step out of the first-person and become a spectator viewing yourself as you run your race. From this vantage point, you can see if you have the correct body position and alignment needed to produce winning results.

4. Now step back once more into the first-person. If necessary, make any mental and physical adjustments needed to enhance your results.

VISUALIZATION

Visualization can be used not only by athletes, but by anyone contemplating a challenging occasion. The businessman who wants to see how he will handle a tough presentation can visualize himself in the first-person delivering his talk. Then he can "listen" from his clients point of view. These techniques are highly effective and will give you the confidence and added edge you need to win. They don't require any particular training or skills, just a strong desire to put forth your best effort and achieve success. At first you may want to try visualizing a short, simple feat, such as a dive into the water, the first steps of a race or the introduction to your speech. When you've mastered that to your satisfaction, you can move on to a scenario which encompasses the entire event.

As with any technique, the more you use it, the more ease you will develop and the more effective it will be. Visualization techniques are sometimes used in a variety of self-actualizing practices, but the principle is simple and easily learned. *So go for it — it's a great "Secret Weapon," used by SUPERSTARS IN ALL FIELDS.*

HERBAL HEALING COMPRESS

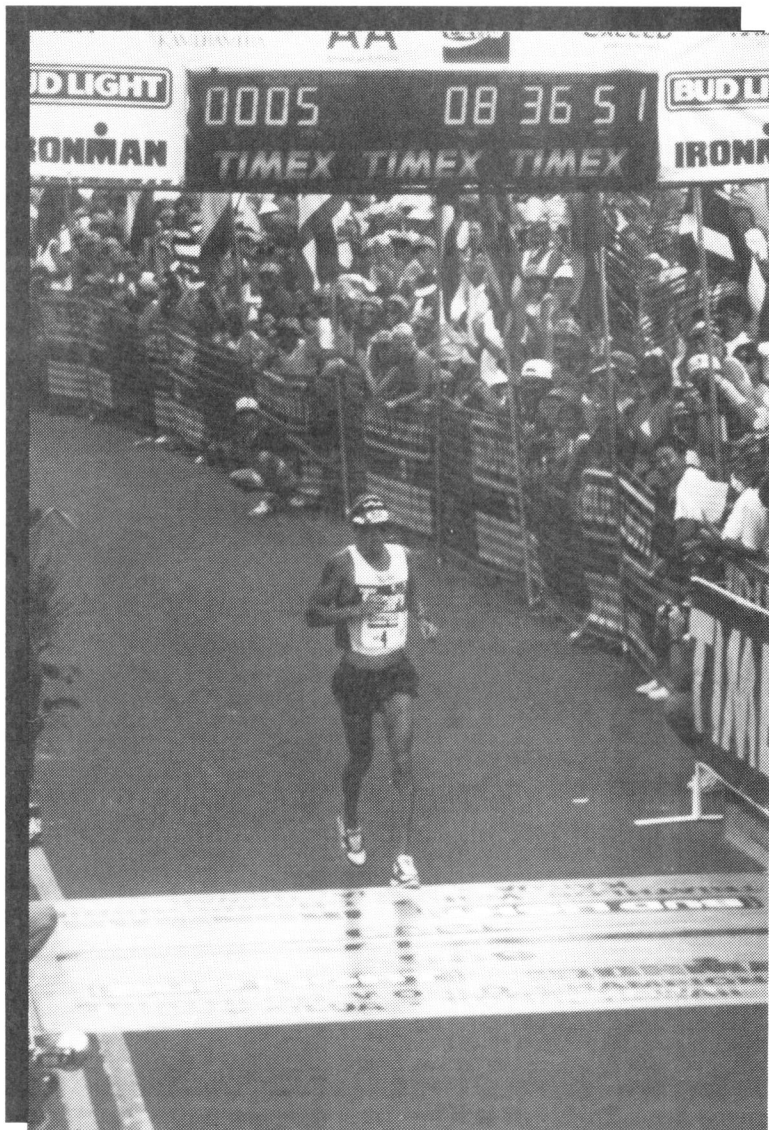

Photo by Russell Moore

Scott Tinley
Ironman
October 14, 1989, Kona, Hawaii

After the Ironman, Scott used my Herbal Healing compress to soak his legs in — which helped to remove the soreness from his legs and speed his recovery.

HERBAL HEALING COMPRESS
Testimonial by John Finch, Herbalist

I first encountered this herbal combination after suffering a painful injury while playing basketball. I visited an M. D. who advised arthoscopic surgery to repair torn ligaments and was told the recovery time could be many months. I then visited our herbalist and friend (also an M. D.), who gave me a bag of roots, barks, and other herbs. A towel was to be soaked in a strong hot tea made with these ingredients. This was to be wrapped around my knee with a hot water bottle on top for 30 minutes or more twice a day. I asked the doctor if this treatment would make my knee feel better, and he replied if would not only make it feel better, but would actually speed the healing process.

I didn't understand how putting something on the outside would heal internal injuries, but decided to give it a try. To my surprise, my knee began to feel better almost immediately and swelling was reduced. Within a few weeks I was walking normally and in only two months, I was back on the basketball court!

The use of a hot compress for injuries with inflammation is counter to current practice in Western medicine. To reduce inflammation, ice is recommended. A cold application however, is just what the injured area does not need. Injury involves a blockage of energy and fluids resulting in a cold local condition. High voltage photography reveals the blue color around injuries indicating the loss of heat in those areas. By further blocking the flow of energy and fluids the healing process is actually retarded. Ice packs also involve a degree of discomfort as the body lets us know how it feels about additional cold at the injured site.

Application of herbal compresses relieves the pain involved in the initial stage of an injury, restores warmth, energy, and fluid circulation (which reduces inflammation naturally), soothes inflamed membranes, relaxes local muscles, disinfects, and promotes a rapid repair process.

I have used the healing compress several times since for ankle and thumb sprains and have recommended it to many friends who report similar experiences. It has also been used to reduce the pain and swelling of arthritis, tendonitis, bruises, and other muscle, tendon, ligament, and bone disorders.

HERBAL HEALING COMPRESS

A COMPRESS (OR FOMENTATION) is the application of heat and moisture to ease pain and reduce inflammation.

INDICATIONS: Pulled muscles, ligaments, tendons; fractures, sprains, wounds (after closing), inflammations, spasms.

DIRECTIONS: Gently simmer 1/2 cup of herbs in 1 quart of water For 45 minutes. A hand, elbow, or foot may be soaked directly in hot tea, reheating as required to maintain maximum tolerable temperature. For knees, shoulders, hips, etc. soak a towel or cloth in tea and apply to affected area as hot as can be tolerated without discomfort, cover with plastic or "Saran Wrap". Place a heating pad or hot water bottle on top. Cover with a dry (flannel) cloth or towel. Generally application should be for at least 30 minutes. After treatment (wring out towel and) refrigerate tea. Repeat 2 or 3 times a day as needed. Tea can be reused for up to a week in this manner.

HYDROTHERAPY: Hot compress (or soak) may be alternated with a shorter application of a cold compress (or ice water soak). Heat serves to relax the body and open the pores. Cold stimulates the body and causes contraction. Alternation between hot and cold will revitalize the affected area.

HERBAL HEALING COMPRESS
INGREDIENTS

INGREDIENTS and their major properties:

BLACK WALNUT LEAVES ....Astringent

CHAPARRAL ....Antiseptic

COMFREY LEAF AND ROOT ....Demulcent, Vulnerary, Astringent

LOBELIA..Antispasmodic

MARSHMALLOW ....Demulcent, Emollient, Vulnerary

MULLEIN LEAF ....Astringent, Vulnerary, Demulcent

SKULLCAP...Antispasmodic

WHITE OAK BARK ....Astringent

WORMWOOD ....Antiseptic

GRAVEL ROOT ....Astringent, Antiseptic, Demulcent

— GLOSSSARY OF PHARMACOLOGICAL TERMS —

Antiseptic: Inhibits growth of micro-organisms.

Antispasmodic: Prevents or eases muscular spasms or convulsions.

Astringent: Causes contraction of tissues, checking the discharge of fluid and mucus. Generally antiseptic.

Demulcent: Soothes inflamed mucus surfaces and protects them from irritation. Cools, coats, and lubricates.

Vulnerary: Curative, promotes cell growth and wound healing.

For more information about how to obtain the Herbal Healing Compress write to:

Sports Touch
P.O. Box 229002-155
San Diego, CA 92122

COMMON SENSE NUTRITION

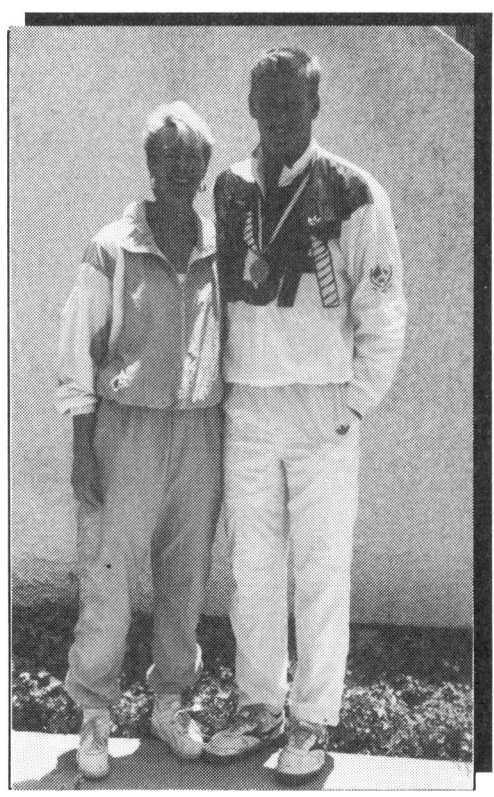

Bob Ctvrtlik and myself

Common Sense. Putting only what is good and healthy into your body enhances strength, stamina, endurance, energy, vitality, mental activity and alertness. This will make you a gold medal winner.

NUTRITION
A COMMON SENSE APPROACH

"Common Sense Nutrition" means exactly that: **Common Sense**. Putting only what is good and healthy into your body enhances strength, stamina, endurance, energy, vitality, mental acuity and alertness. Assuming, of course, that you don't counter-balance those nutrients with unhealthy substances. Cigarettes, drugs and excessive alcohol decrease your longevity, compromise your immune system and make you susceptible to a host of disorders. But with a properly fueled, healthy body, you should wake-up each day feeling refreshed and ready for challenges.

Guidelines for good nutrition are basically the same for everyone. But because athletes expend an unusual amount of energy, they require more nutrients than a less active person. However, the **quality** of those nutrients is just as important as the **quanity**.

COMMON SENSE NUTRITION
GUIDELINES

Guidelines for "Common Sense Nutrition" and a longer and more productive life are as follows:

1. Get approximately 8 hours of sleep every night.

2. Drink approximately 8-10, 8 oz. glasses of water each day. (Your body is approx. 80% water. It needs constant replenishment to prevent dehydration.)

3. Eat plenty of fresh, raw organic fruits and vegetables (without pesticides or other chemicals).

4. Eat enough meat, poultry, fish, grains and vegetables to provide ample protein for your body. Protein is essential for maintenance and repair of muscle tissue.

5. Because most of us experience stress in both our professional and personal lives, it might be a good idea to enhance your diet with a good multiple vitamin and mineral supplement.

6. If you are a competitive athlete, you may need to eat six small meals a day, so as not to deplete your energy reserves.

7. If you are a competitive athlete, you should also *select one day each week for rest.* Get off your feet and relax! This helps your body to heal and recuperate, while allowing your mind to unwind and take a break.

8. Get a massage !

   Touching is a necessity, not a luxury, and most of us don't get touched often enough. A good massage will make you feel wonderful as it relieves stress and tension in your muscles, and gets rid of those "knots" in your shoulders, neck, head and back.

   As an athlete, regular massage is a must, for it speeds recovery time. "The sooner an athlete can get back on the court, the more productive he will be for himself and his team." *Bob Ctvrtlik, USA Volleyball, 1988.*

COMMON SENSE NUTRITION
GUIDELINES (cont'd)

9. Meditation - Stress is a major contributor to both physical illness and mental and emotional distress. One of the best ways to combat it is to find a quite place each day, where you can relax without distractions. Then close your eyes and meditate on your health and well-being.

    When your body is free of stress, your digestion and elimination system works better. This exercise will leave you feeling refreshed and with more energy to start or continue your day.

10. Declare A Holidax!* Allow yourself the time to get away from it all at least once or twice a year for a week or longer, and treat yourself to weekend getaways whenever possible.

    These change-of-scenes and routines invigorate and relax us at the same time. If you can't afford a jaunt with the Jet Set, don't worry — the world is rich with opportunities, and not all of them come with a high price tag. Museums, parks, beaches, and mountains are all public domain and with a little creativity you can plan excursions that lift your spirits without ravaging your wallet.

11. SMILE and LAUGH a lot! A wide range of studies have shown that laughter is indeed the best medicine — a gift that will keep you young. This top-of-the- line stressbuster, along with a positive outlook goes along way towards promoting good health as well as happiness.

    Be good to yourself. Treat your body (as you do your car) like a beautifully constructed physical machine. It can last along time if you give it the right fuel, massage it regularly (oil and lube), and allow it proper rest. Proper maintenance will increase your "mileage" and insure life-long top performance!

*   *Holiday + Relax = Holidax*

SPORTS INJURIES AND ACCIDENTS

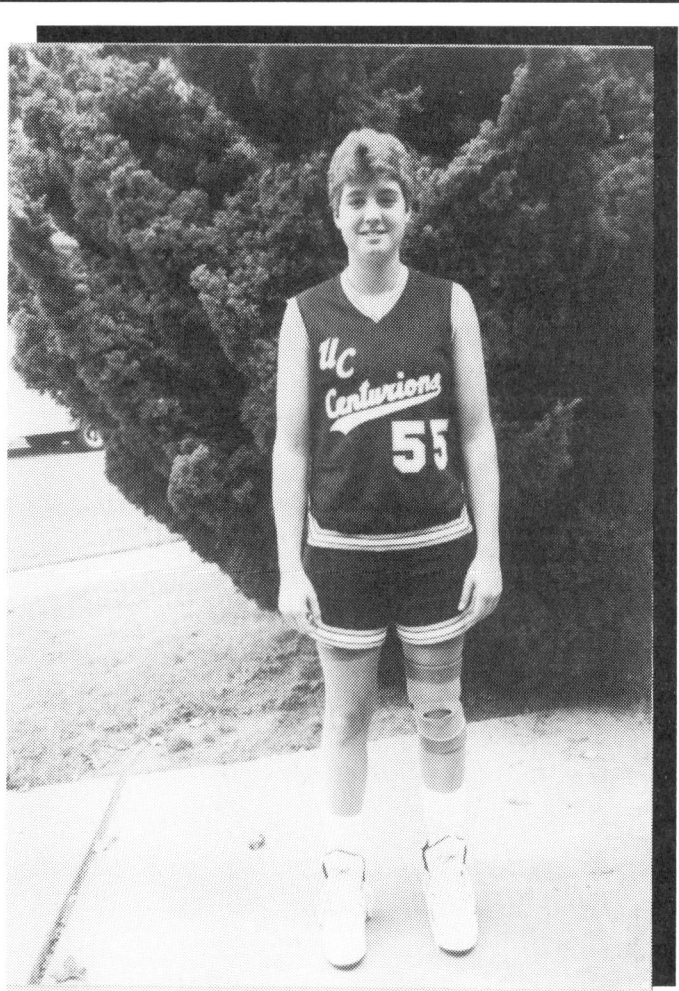

Charlotte Kornik

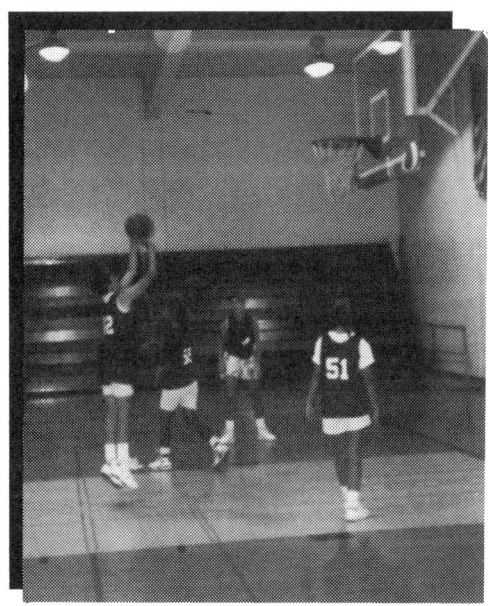

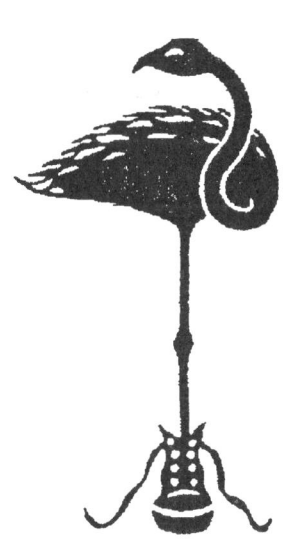

SPORTS INJURIES AND ACCIDENTS

What You Can Do Immediately After An Injury:

As an athlete at any level, in any sport, there are bound to be injuries of various magnitude. We all say, "It won't happen to me," but in sports and in life, there are no guarantees. Whether it's riding a bike, running or even walking, you can twist your ankle, take a tumble, or get hit by a ball. And do you know what is the very first thing that happens when we suffer a blow or a jolt of any kind? Although you're not aware of it, you momentarily stop breathing!

The body goes into a temporary form of shock when this most basic rhythm is thrown out-of-balance. When it happens, the body's internal rhythm is interrupted for a split second and has to start up again. And it doesn't always return immediately to its original state.

We all have our own biological time clock. Some people are more aware of their personal rhythm than others, and are very tuned into what feels "right" and what doesn't.

Diaphragmatic breathing, pg. 10 along with the Sports Touch Energy Balancing. pg. 37 – 44 are two of the ways to help reset your body's delicate and natural time clock and return your system to normal as quickly as possible.

By immediately starting diaphragmatic breathing, you will feel more relaxed, calm and able to think more clearly. Depending on the seriousness of an injury, you will need to make sure your structure is in alignment. You may then need to seek professional help from a medical doctor, chiropractor, osteopath, or acupuncturist in order to regain a full and proper balance of your vital energy. For scrapes, bruises and swelling, I recommend my Herbal Healing Compress, pg. 87 – 88 and the use of oral homeopathics; such as ARNICA MONTANA 30C, which aids in bruising and muscular aches; and RUTA GRAVEOLENS 6C, which aids in the healing of ligaments. Until you receive professional help for more serious injuries, do the Sports Touch Ritual and Energy Balancing, pg. 37 – 44.

Those actions will immediately start your body on its road to recovery. Time is of the essence, so don't delay — take action as soon as you possibly can.

SPORTS INJURIES
OVER TRAINING

When I arrived in Kona for the Ironman, I saw many athletes out running and cycling, still training, most of them were not really resting and hydrating as I thought they would be. This lack of care can lead to over-training and injuries. Once you have spent months getting yourself physically and mentally prepared for a race as important as the Ironman, or any other ultra-endurance event, when the time actually comes around, it's too late for last minute heroic efforts.

Two weeks before the event you should be toning down and doing a bare minimum of training. You also need to hydrate yourself by drinking lots of water, resting, stretching and mentally visualizing how you will put forth your best effort. It's important to eat the proper food to nourish and fuel your body and to give it that extra measure of stamina and endurance.

Going for a mile swim to stretch out is great, or you might choose to run a mile or two, but remember, in the heat of the Kona sun, you will quickly dehydrate, so be aware and keep the water flowing.

The final week before the event is rough, and tensions are understandably high. But the big day is close at hand and you want to be in the best possible condition and ready to cut loose with an optimum performance!

TESTIMONIAL
SPORTS INJURIES

Charlotte Kornik, age 16, Junior at University City High School Varsity Girls Basketball Team, in San Diego, California.

"On December 14, 1989, I was participating in a High School Basketball game. In the last forty-eight seconds of the game, I went up for a rebound and subsequently came down on my ankle. It was a bad sprain.

"The hour following the game, Kate took me to her home and applied the Herbal Compress directly on my ankle. She also gave me homeopathic pellets to minimize the bruising and allow my body to heal naturally. The homeopathic pellets were ARNICA MONTANA 30C, which aids in bruising and muscular aches and RUTA GRANEOLENS 6C, which aids in the healing of ligaments.

"Within one hour, the swelling was completely gone and I was able to begin small movements. I continued to apply the herbs to my ankle every hour for thirty minutes till bedtime.

"The next day, I again continued the Herbal Compress on my ankle and homeopathics the entire day. When I administered the Herbs, I started slow movements which increased blood flow and kept my flexibility. During these two days, I stayed completely off the ankle.

"By the third day, I noticed a significant change in my ankle. I was able to put fifty percent of my full weight on my ankle — but I continued to stay off of it and apply herbs hourly, continued movement of the ankle and the homeopathics.

"By day four, I was walking on my ankle, doing exercises, but keeping my activity to a minimum so as to allow the tendons and muscles to heal. I used the herbs every two — three hours and continued the homeopathics.

"By the sixth day, I was able to put full weight on my ankle and resume normal activity. I did attend basketball practice but only to practice shooting. I did not play for almost a week later.

"Such a common injury would have resulted in being laid-up for two — three weeks. However, thanks to Kate's program of the Herbal Compress, Homeopathics, Light Massage, Slow Movement-Exercises, and Rest, I overcame an injury in approximately four days!

"I am very thankful for finding Kate and I will never doubt her techniques again! They really do work! My coach, and teammates thank you too, Kate."

ALTERNATIVE THERAPIES

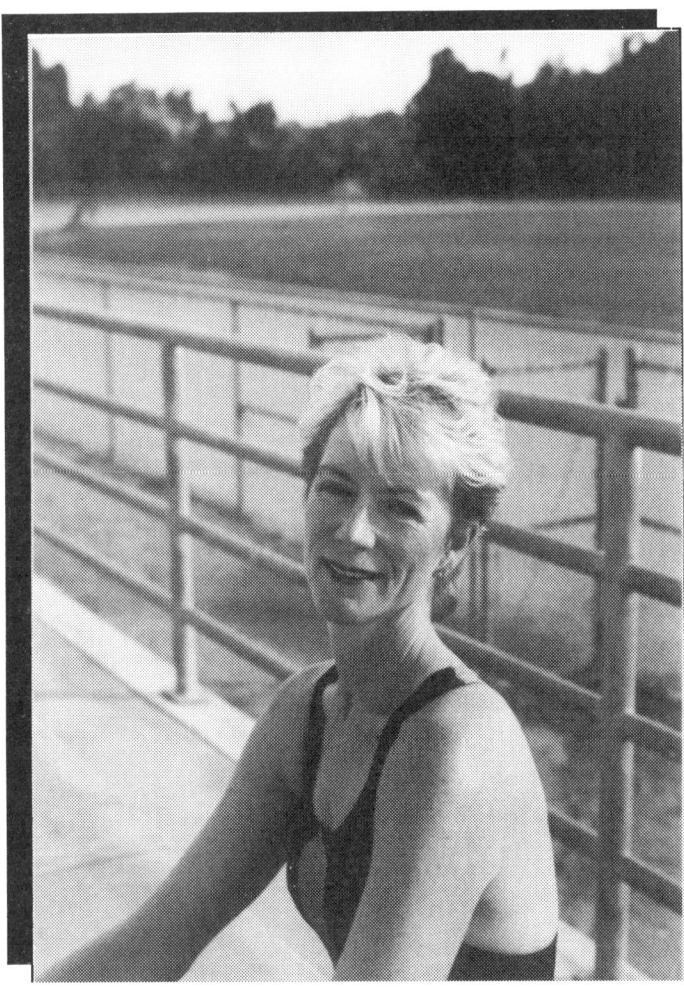

Kate Montgomery
Certified Sports Massage Therapist

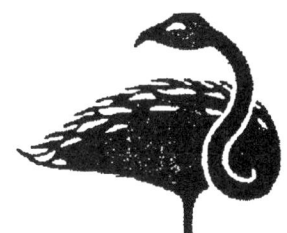

Although Alternative Health Care Practioners can benefit you during times of illness or injury, they are also valuable in the area of prevention... which, of course, is the best "Remedy" of all.

ALTERNATIVE THERAPIES

Chiropractic, Massage, Acupuncture

All three of these alternative therapies can be used in conjunction with one another and also with traditional therapies. It's up to you to take charge of your health care, for no one else has the awareness necessary to determine the proper course for you.

Don't be afraid to try these alternative methods, and see how they work. And remember, there are as many different Chiropractors, Massage Therapists, and Acupuncturists as there are medical doctors, and they vary widely in terms of expertise, emphasis and personal style.

RESPONSIBILITY

It is your responsibility and yours alone to seek out the best possible health care for yourself and your family. It's up to you to ask questions and set-up as many consultations as necessary until you are satisfied with the answers. As part of your overall health program, you may wish to explore the benefits of Alternative Health Care. Also known as Preventive Medicine. Three such therapies are Acupuncture, Chiropractic and Massage Therapy.

The reason I'm discussing these therapies is because I feel most people lack a clear understanding of how and why and when to use these treatments. The main thing to remember is this: Although Alternative Health Care Practioners can benefit you during times of illness or injury, they are also valuable in the area of prevention... which, of course is the best "Remedy" of all.

ALTERNATIVE THERAPIES
REGULAR MASSAGE

Why is it important to have REGULAR MASSAGE?

STRESS!!! Stress is the number one cause of sore, tight shoulders, low-back pain, headaches, and then injuries caused by accidents. If you are an athlete or weekend warrior, you have a special need for massage therapy.

For just a moment, think of your body as a car. You're probably quite conscientious about changing your auto's oil, spark plugs, and check the water in the battery. You likely wash and wax it every week. So why not do the same for your body to keep it running in prime condition. Those sore muscles you complain about are caused by waste products, poisons and toxins, harmful chemical by-products caused by exercise. During exercise you tear micro-fibers in the muscles creating "ropey" muscles that can restrict your flexibility and movement.

A massage readily eliminates all these discomforts and with proper massage, recovery time is shortened. A healthy body should not have pain... it's not something you have to live with or should grow accustomed to. A deep massage once a week or twice a month is the best preventive therapy, as it protects you from developing a host of pains and disorders.

Not only does massage relax the body, but it also revitalizes the mind. With regular massage you'll find that your mental attitude will begin to change. Life will start looking and feeling wonderfully different. If you make your body a priority and treat it with the same regard you have for your car, it will last longer and feel infinitely better! And although I hesitate to make any "fountain-of-youth" claims, most massage recipients find themselves looking and feeling significantly younger. Living proof of this is Bess James, a 79 year young client who climbed the Pikes Peak Ascent in 1988 and runs 2-3 marathons a year and numerous 10K's.

ALTERNATIVE THERAPIES
MASSAGE THERAPY

Education for a Massage Therapist:

1. Graduate from a 500-1000 hour accredited massage school.

2. Carry malpractice insurance.

3. Belong to a professional organization such as the American Massage Association, American Professional Massage Therapists and Bodyworkers, International Mysmassethics Federation, Inc., California Health Practioners Association, to name a few.

4. Continuing classes in the profession.

There are a number of different types of massage therapy, each with its own purpose. **Swedish massage** - for relaxation; **Lymphatic massage** - removal of poisons and toxins from the system - a very light massage; **Shiatsu, Japanese acupressure massage** - pressing various energy points along an energy pathway to restore the vital energy of the body; **Trager - movement massage** to establish better flexibility; **Rolfing** - is not massage, but a form of structural realignment of the muscles; **Sports Massage** - offers pre-event, post-event, training massage, rehabilitative massage for the athlete and many more.

These are not merely types of massage but forms of structural and flexibility changes and releases. And just as you would take care in choosing a physician, it's wise to prudently select a massage therapist. Don't hesitate to inquire about his/her background, and ask detailed questions about training and length and type of experience. The right person will not be offended but rather will welcome your questions and answer them to your satisfaction.

To find a qualified massage therapist/practioner, use the list I have provided in Appendix III, pg. 149 – 150. These are only a few of the many organizations in this country. You can call these organizations to find someone in your area. Ask friends to recommend someone they use. "Word of mouth" is almost always the best way to find a qualified therapist.

SPORTS MASSAGE

Sports Massage should be an integral part of every athlete's training program. It's important to learn about pre-event, post-event, and training or rehabilitative massage techniques which can enhance both your training and your performance in competitions.

Exercise is good for us, however, exercise can stress and strain the muscle tissue. It can injure the tendons and ligaments, which are frequently stretched beyond their normal bounds. As we exercise or compete we are setting the stage for muscle damage and soreness. For example: when we run, our leg muscles are going through repetitive contractions which create microscopic tears in the muscle fibers. This brings about pain and can lead to inflammation and more pain. Muscle soreness immediately after a training session or event is due to a build-up of metabolic by-products such as lactic acid and a lack of oxygen (ischemia) to the muscle tissue. This lack of oxygen to the muscle tissue and build-up of waste by-products (poisons and toxins) causes pain which can cause a muscle spasm. Our muscles become hard, inflexible, and ropey - adhesions that build-up over a period of years.

MASSAGE TO THE RESCUE! WHAT CAN IT DO FOR YOU?

Massage reaches these exercise-damaged muscles. Done properly, the deep massage stimulates circulation, increases lymphatic flow, breaks up fibrosis that binds and glues one muscle fiber to another, relaxes muscle spasms and relieves pain.

SPORTS MASSAGE

HOW DOES MASSAGE WORK?

By kneading, rolling and stretching muscle tissue, we are able to lubricate and clean the muscles via the lymphatic system. Lymph is known as the "motor oil" of the human body. It decreases friction between the muscles and aids in the removal of lactic acid and other harmful waste by-products caused by exertion.

Massage increases the effectiveness of blood circulation and the best possible state of nutrition to the muscles. It helps to break up scar tissue, loosens muscle fibers by separating them from one another so they can act freely, with more flexibility. It helps to lengthen muscles shortened by frequent and hard contractions of athletes. Thus eliminating fatigue, promoting relaxation, reduces muscle tension, relieves swelling and helps cut your recovery time to practically nothing.

SPORTS MASSAGE

Sports Massage recognizes that you have different needs at different times. Four different kinds of Sports Massage are...

PRE-EVENT

A quick treatment that will be an adjunct to your warm-up. It consists of COMPRESSION STROKES — a rhythmic pumping on the muscle to create a sustained increase in circulation and muscle relaxation. Pumping on a muscle will double blood volume and hold it for 40 minutes — Russian sports massage interpreted by Dr. Michael Yessiss. JOSTLING of the muscles to excite the nerve endings so they remain alert. CROSS FIBER FRICTION to the origins and insertions of the muscles warming the muscles tendons.

All of these massage techniques can be done by the athlete.

POST-EVENT

A light massage that will increase your circulation and lymphatic flow to speed the removal of toxins, relieve muscle spasms and prevent soreness. This massage is calming to the nervous system and relaxing to the mind.

TRAINING MASSAGE

This massage is used for regular fine tuning. It is used as a "search and destroy" mission to relieve the biomechanical stresses in your muscles before they become a problem. By doing this massage on a regular basis, you will be able to train harder and more consistently.

REHABILITATIVE MASSAGE

This type of massage is done when you have incurred an injury. It will speed your healing, increase your range of motion and create a scar that is strong but allows the muscle to broaden normally.

PREVENTION is the key to athletic performance. Keeping the athlete actively training in a supple condition is the major goal of sports massage. No one likes to have conditions such as achilles tendonitis, shin splints or hamstring problems that can escalate and cause serious damage. Massage is NOT a luxury, it should be an integral part of every athlete's training program, and very likely will be the best investment you'll ever make!

ALTERNATIVE THERAPIES
CHIROPRACTIC

Why do you need a Chiropractor?

A Chiropractor is a specialist who can help keep your skeleton properly aligned. For when the skeleton is out of alignment, an assortment of problems can result, from headaches, insomnia and incontinence, to pain and numbness and this directly affects the function of organs and muscles.

As children and young adults, most of us grew up falling off bicycles, playground equipment, playing contact sports (football, soccer, wrestling etc..) and generally getting into rough-and-tumble situations. These long forgotten injuries can recur in the form of low-back pain, shoulder pain, and neck pain years down the road. And maintenance is the key to avoiding them. Ideally, such maintenance should begin in childhood to head off back problems before they take hold and become troublesome later in life.

Once you are an adult, maintenance is the only way to stabilizing your spine and keeping it healthy and free of pain.

ALTERNATIVE THERAPIES
EDUCATION FOR A CHIROPRACTOR

Most people are not aware of the education a Doctor of Chiropractor receives. A doctor of chiropractic attends six years of college — two years pre-professional plus four years professional. A comparison of classes attended by a Doctor of Chiropractic versus a Medical Doctor are as follows:

MEDICAL Class Hours (Minimum)	AND Subject	CHIROPRACTIC Class Hours (Minimum)
508	Anatomy	520
326	Physiology	420
335	Pathology	271
325	Chemistry	300
130	Bacteriology	114
374	Diagnosis	370
112	Neurology	320
148	X-Ray	217
144	Psychiatry	65
198	Obstetrics & Gynecology	65
156	Orthopedics	225
,756	TOTAL HOURS	2,887

Plus, classes in Adjusting, Manipulation, Kinesiology, and other similar subjects related to his specialty. A total of 4,485 hrs. A medical doctor receives a total of 4,248 classroom hours. As you can see, a Doctor of Chiropractic is a highly qualified professional.

ALTERNATIVE THERAPIES
ACUPUNCTURE – Chinese Therapy

Acupuncture has been used for centuries by the Chinese. This practice treats the body as a whole, not just as isolated parts. You may be experiencing headaches but have no clue as to their basic cause. An Acupuncturist will evaluate your entire body and discover pertinent facts about your digestive system, your mental attitude, your sleeping patterns, skin temperature, etc... All these observations help him in determining the best treatment for your particular problem. If your energy or "battery" has run down and needs recharging an acupuncturist can raise your energy level , relieve pain and discomfort and bring your vital energy back into balance. Promoting and maintaining better overall health.

Acupuncture consists of using needles to stimulate points along an energy pathway called a meridian. The use of herbs in Chinese medicine is used predominantly in China, but is making its way into the United States as well, as a way to help regulate and build the body's defenses against disease.

ALTERNATIVE THERAPIES
ACUPUNCTURE – Education

A student of acupuncture attends school for 3 years. Classes consists of:

Anatomy	Acupuncture Theory	
Physiology	pathology/Treatment	
Neurology	Diagnosis/Evaluation	
Physiopathology	point location	
Biology	needling	
Biochemistry	Other techniques	
Bio-physics	Herbology	
Clinical Diagnosis		
Homeopathic	Qi Gong	Counseling
Nutrition	Tai Qi	

What to look for when considering an Acupuncturist:

1. Background/school
2. How long in practice
3. What is his specialty - types of problems he deals with
4. Personality of the doctor
5. What areas of Oriental Medicine is the doctor most versed in.
   a. Needling
   b. Herbology
   c. Nutrition
   d. Exercise Therapy (Qi Gong)
   e. Pediatrics/Gyn.
   f. Is there a psychology/counseling background

A Doctor of Acupuncture is a highly qualified professional. The methods may seem a lot different from western-style diagnostic techniques but they are complete and efficient getting to the bottom of the dis-ease.

APPENDIX I – EXTRA TIPS

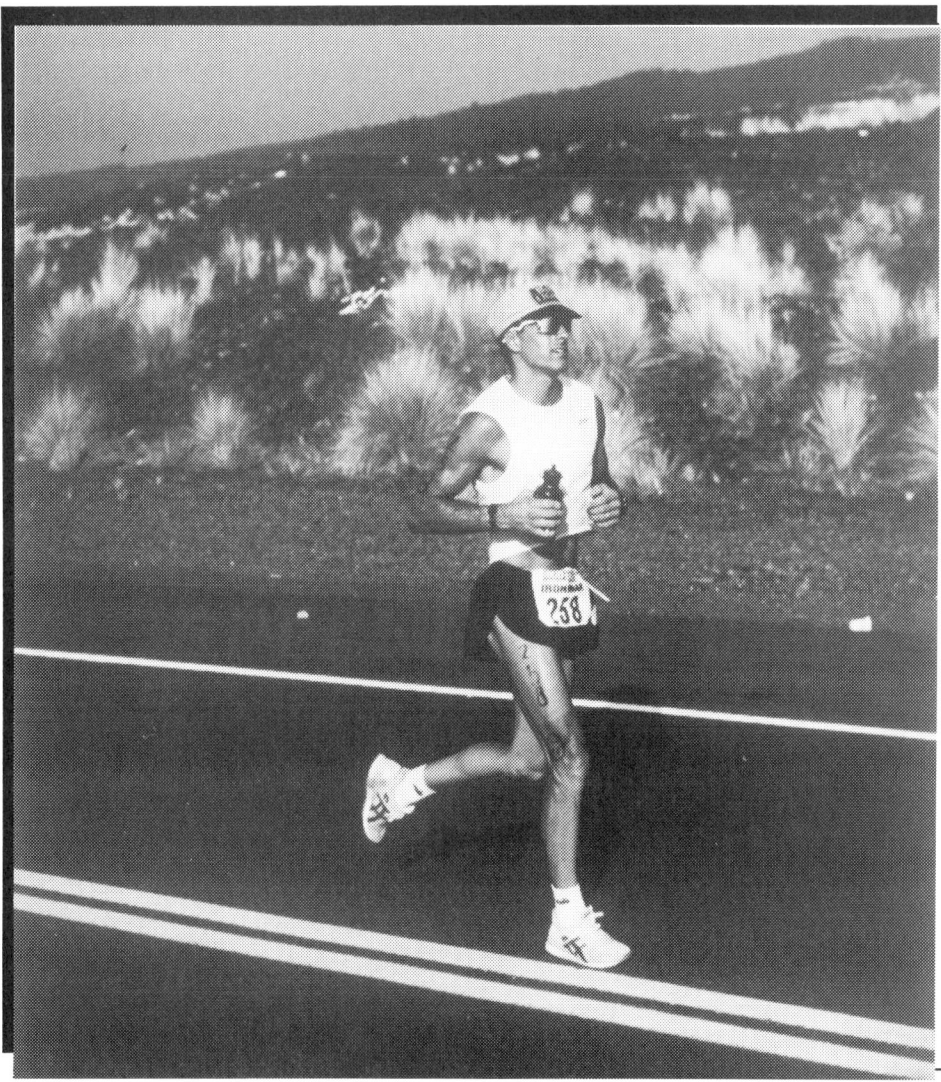

"I was experiencing lower-back pain and you showed me where to apply pressure. I did this prior to race day and never experienced the back pain that was so difficult to deal with in training."

— **John Carey**
Triathlete
Canada

(Refer to Tip #I.)

EXTRA TIPS

I.   Lower back muscle - Quadratus lumborum, as pictured below. Standing, find the end of the rib cage. Place thumbs under the last rib, press into the spine. If sore, the muscle is in spasm or has a trigger point. A trigger point is a hyper-sensitive area that refuses to lenghten - caused by overuse, injury, or emotional trauma. Work your way down , pressing into the spine, until you reach the top of the hip. Hold each point for at least 90 sec.or until the pain subsides. Afterwards do side-bends to stretch this muscle (as pictured on pg. 76). Do slowly. Diaphragmatically breathe through this whole process.

II.   To loosen and relax shoulders: Take the opposite hand to the opposite shoulder - grab hold of the shoulder muscle, (Trapezius m.), lean over to the side and shake the arm hanging down. Do the opposite shoulder. Repeat as needed to relax shoulders.

III.   Do shoulder shrugs to relax the muscles of the shoulders and upper back. Raise shoulders to ears and back down.

IV.   Take a hot Epsom Salts bath (2 cups) for 15 minutes. Epsom Salts helps to draw waste products such as lactic acid from sore and tired muscles. *Bathe only after competition or a hard day of training – never within 24 hours prior to competition. This can make you very "sluggish" and slow you down for your competition.

*   **If you are sore 24 hours prior to competition, take a 5 minute epsom salts bath only.**

V.   Drink at least 8 - 10 glasses of water each day and more when training.

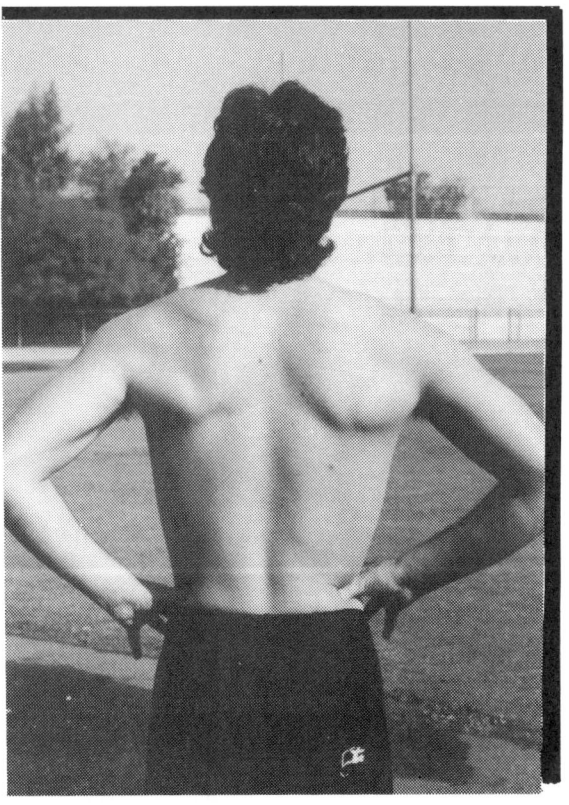

APPENDIX II – SAMPLE RITUALS

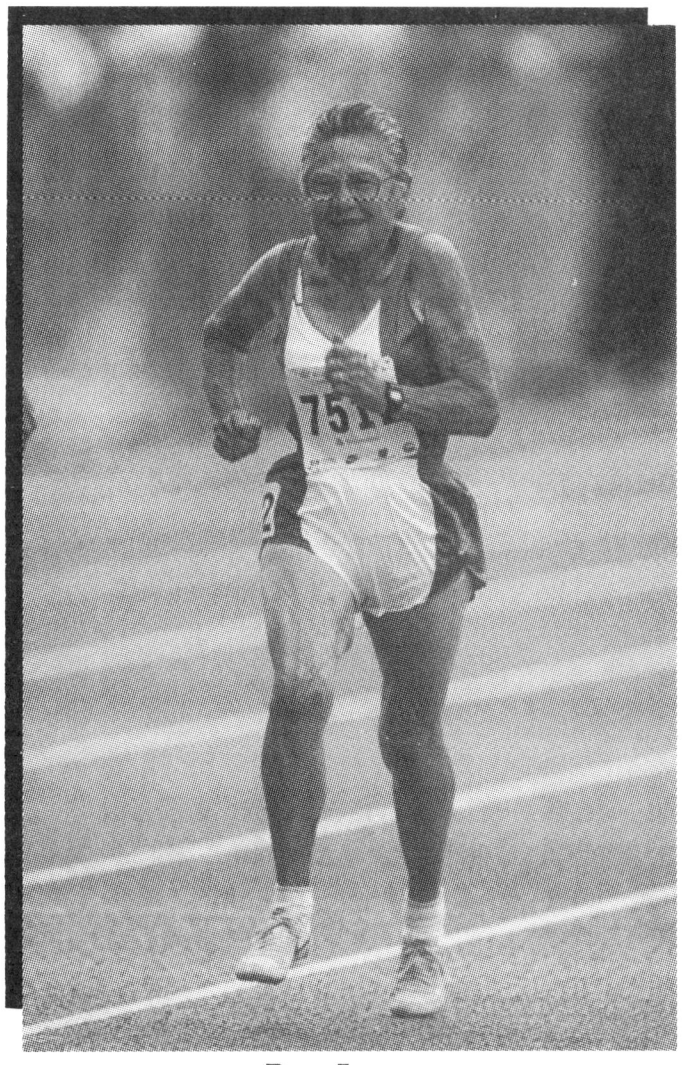

Bess James
79 years old
Masters Runner
Holder of World and
American Records

"While climbing Pike's Peak, I concentrated on Diaphragmatic Breathing as Kate taught me, rubbing my neuro-lymphatic points constantly. When I reached the top, I felt great and wasn't even tired."

SAMPLE RITUALS

Steps one, three, four and five of the ritual should be done as a preventive, daily, to ensure your vital energy level stays high and balanced. Step two — when training or competing.

Prelude to all rituals:

1. Wake up in the morning and breathe diaphragmatically ten times. (Refer to pg. 10.)

2. Diaphragm release. (Refer to pg. 22.)

3. Get out of bed and sit on the floor (hard surface) and rock on your sacrum — the Sacral Rock. (Refer to pg. 30 – 31.)

4. Respiratory Spinal Extension — stretches the back muscles. (Refer to pg. 32 – 33.)

5. Two-Minute Energy Balance. (Refer to pg. 35 – 44.)

6. Warm-up at least 5 – 10 minutes prior to stretching to get blood into muscles. NEVER STRETCH COLD.

7. Add stretching before and after a competition or training session. (Refer to pg. 62 – 78 for more about stretching.)

8. Add visualization to your training sessions. (Refer to pg. 83 – 84 on how.)

Once you have done these steps, you are ready to select neuro-lymphatic points and acupressure points to be used in your training and competitive programs.

SAMPLE RITUALS
DAILY RITUAL

A daily ritual could consist of these steps:

MORNING

1. Wake up in the morning and breathe diaphragmatically ten times.

2. Diaphragm release, if necessary.

3. Get out of bed and sit on the floor (hard surface) and rock on your sacrum — the Sacral Rock.

4. Respiratory Spinal Extension — stretches the back muscles and resets the sacrum.

5. Two-Minute Energy Balance.

6. Acupressure points — **PUMP FIRMLY**.

Lg. I. 4	Stimulates the immune system; moves blood and Qi
St. 36	Stimulates the immune system; increases vitality
Spl. 6	Stimulates the immune system
T.W. 5	Stimulates the immune system
C.V. 17	Stimulates respirations; releases Qi and emotions
T.W. 4	Increases energy
T.W. 23	Harmonizes the body — **HOLD LIGHTLY**

7. Stretch using the twelve basic stretches introduced in this book.

8. Proceed on with your exercise routine and remember to stretch afterwards.

HAVE A GREAT DAY!

— KATE

SAMPLE RITUALS
SPRINTER

DAILY

1. Diaphragm breathing - 10 times
2. Diaphragm Release
3. Sacral Rock
4. Respiratory spinal extension
5. Two-Minute Energy Balance
6. Warm-up for 5 minutes (jumping jacks) and stretch for 30 minutes
7. Visualize the event

PRE-RACE

1. Pre-oxygenate - Diaphragmatically breathe as much as you can 10-20 minutes before competition.
2. Acupressure points - **PUMP FIRMLY**

Lg.I. 4	T.W. 4	C.V. 17
Lg.I. 10	St. 36	K. 3

3. Neuro-Lymphatics - **RUB FIRMLY**

    Diaphragm

    Quadriceps
4. Neuro-vasculars - hold lightly

    Hand behind knee - warms up muscle behind knee

POST RACE

1. Warm down.   Then do COOL DOWN ACUPRESSURE POINTS.
2. Neuro-lymphatics **RUB FIRMLY**

Quadriceps	Buttock muscles (glutes)
Hamstrings	Diaphragm

3. That night take a Hot Epsom Salts Bath to relax the muscles.
4. Drink a lot of water.
5. Get plenty of rest.
6. Stretch for 30 minutes, hold each position for 1 minute.
7. Get a massage.

SAMPLE RITUALS
ENDURANCE RUNNER

DAILY

1. Diaphragm Breathing - 10 times
2. Diaphragm Release
3. Sacral Rock
4. Respiratory Spinal Extension
5. Two-Minute Energy Balance
6. Warm-up 5 minutes (jumping jacks) and stretch 30 minutes
7. Visualize the event

PRE-RACE

1. Pre-oxygenate your lungs as much as possible
2. Acupressure Points, **PUMP FIRMLY** 10-20 minutes prior to the event.

Lg.I. 4	T.W. 4	K. 3
Lg.I. 10	C.V. 17	St. 36

3. Neuro-lymphatics - **RUB FIRMLY** after warm-up. 10-20 minutes prior to the race.

   Quadriceps   Psoas - drink water and rub this point
   Diaphragm

DURING RACE

1. Acupressure Points, **PUMP FIRMLY** every 1 - 2 miles

Lg.I. 4	C.V. 17
Lg.I. 10	

2. **Neuro-lymphatics - RUB FIRMLY as much as possible during the run.**
   Diaphragm
   Quadriceps

SAMPLE RITUALS

ENDURANCE RUNNER

POST RACE

1. Warm down , then do COOL DOWN POINTS AND CONTINUE TO RUB NEURO-LYMPHATICS TO FACILITATE WASH OUT OF TOXINS AND POISONS THAT BUILD UP FROM EXERCISE.

2. That night take a HOT EPSOM SALTS BATH to relax the muscles.

3. Drink plenty of water.

4. Get plenty of rest.

5. Stretch for 30 minutes, hold each position for 1 minute.

6. Get a massage.

SAMPLE RITUALS
TRIATHLON — IRONMAN DISTANCE

DAILY

1. Diaphragm breathing - ten times

2. Diaphragm Release

3. Sacral Rock

4. Respiratory Spinal Extension

5. Two-Minute Energy Balance

6. Warm-up 5 minutes (Jumping Jacks) and stretch 30 minutes

7. Visualize the event

PRE-RACE - SWIM

1. Pre-oxygenate your lungs as much as possible. Deep Diaphragmatic Breaths.

2. Acupressure Points, **PUMP FIRMLY.**

Lg.I. 4	T.W. 4	St. 36
Lg.I. 10	C.V. 17	K. 3

3. Neuro-Lymphatics - Rub firmly

    Diaphragm

    Quadriceps

    arms   - concentrate here for swim, especially
    when the WATER IS COLD.

SWIM TO BIKE TRANSITION

1. Diaphragm Breathing   * Eliminate if going for speed

2. Sacral Rock

3. Respiratory Spinal Extension

BIKE

1. Neuro-lymphatics, **RUB FIRMLY**

    Quadriceps

    Diaphragm

    Supraspinatus   - arm points, rub especially
    after a cold swim

2. Eat and drink plenty of water.

SAMPLE RITUALS
TRIATHLON — IRONMAN DISTANCE

BIKE TO RUN TRANSITION

1. Diaphragm Breathing   * Eliminate if going for speed
2. Rock on the Sacrum
3. Respiratory Spinal Extension

RUN

1. Neuro-lymphatics, **RUB FIRMLY** as much as possible during the run.
    Quadriceps
    Diaphragm
2. Acupressure Points , **PUMP FIRMLY**
    Lg. I. 4   Lg. I. 10
    C.V. 17

DO EVERYTHING EVERY 1 - 2 MILES. Keep breathing and drink plenty water

FOR SPEED IN THE RUN

1. RUB ONLY NEURO-LYMPHATICS FOR THE QUADRICEPS AND DIAPHRAGM
2. PUMP ACUPRESSURE POINT LG. I. 4.

POST-RACE

1. Get checked out by the medical tent if you need to.
2. GET A MASSAGE!
3. Continue to drink plenty of water.
4. Rub neuro-lymphatics for the quadriceps
5. Hold COOL DOWN POINTS.
6. Take a hot EPSOM SALTS BATH OR AN HERBAL HEALING COMPRESS BATH.
7. Stretch for 30 minutes, holding each position for one minute.

SAMPLE RITUALS
CYCLIST

DAILY

1. Diaphragm Breathe - 10 times
2. Diaphragm Release - as needed
3. Sacral Rock
4. Respiratory Spinal Extension
5. Two-Minute Energy Balance
6. Visualize the race

PRE-RACE OR TRAINING

1. Warm-up 5-10 minutes and then stretch for 30 minutes prior to competition or training
2. Race - Pre-oxygenate lungs as much as possible
3. Release trigger points in low-back, (refer to pg. 110, Extra Tips 1) Stretch low-back afterwards doing side bends.
4. Acupressure Points - **PUMP FIRMLY**

Lg.I. 4	T.W. 4	St. 36
Lg.I. 10	C.V. 17	K. 3

5. Neuro-Lymphatic Points - **RUB FIRMLY**

   After warm-up 5-10 minutes prior to competition or training

Diaphragm	Hamstrings
Quadriceps	Low-Back
Psoas	Calves

6. Neuro-Vasculars - **HOLD LIGHTLY**

   Knee - Hold hands lightly behind knee for 30 seconds to 1 minute (Infuses muscles with blood)

7. Massage warm-up

   Rub vigorously sides of knees (medial and lateral collateral ligaments) and above and below the knee cap (quadricep tendon)

SAMPLE RITUALS

CYCLIST

POST-RACE

1. Warm-down and stretch for 30 minutes, holding each position 1 minute
2. Acupressure **COOL DOWN POINTS**
3. Neuro-Lymphatic points
   Quadriceps
   Hamstrings   Low-Back
   Calves   Psoas
4. That night take a **HOT EPSOM SALTS BATH** to relax muscles
5. Drink plenty of water
6. Get plenty of rest
7. Get a massage
   Stretch out your low-back and release any trigger points

SAMPLE RITUALS
SWIMMER

DAILY

1. Diaphragm Breathing - 10 times
2. Diaphragm Release - important to add in
3. Sacral Rock
4. Respiratory Spinal Extension
5. Two-Minute Energy Balance
6. Warm-up for 5 minutes (jumping jacks) and stretch 30 minutes
7. Visualize the event

PRE-RACE

1. Pre-oxygenate your lungs - Diaphragmatically Breathe as much as possible.
2. Acupressure Points, **PUMP FIRMLY** 10-20 minutes prior to the event

Lg.I. 4	C.V. 17
Lg.I. 10	K. 3
T.W. 4	St. 36

3. Neuro-lymphatics - **RUB FIRMLY** after warm-up, 10-20 minutes prior to the race.

Diaphragm	Hamstrings	Neck Flexors and extensors
Arms	Low back	
Quadriceps	Pectorals	
Buttock muscles	Latissimus Dorsi	

   Choose the neuro-lymphatic points that would benefit you the most.

POST RACE

1. Warm down in the pool. Then do COOL DOWN ACUPRESSURE POINTS AND CONTINUE TO RUB NEURO-LYMPHATIC POINTS TO FACILITATE WASH OUT OF TOXINS AND POISONS THAT BUILD UP FROM EXERCISE.
2. That night take a HOT EPSOM SALTS BATH to relax the muscles.
3. Drink plenty of water.
4. Get plenty of rest.
5. Stretch for 30 minutes, holding each position for 1 minute.
6. Get a massage.

SAMPLE RITUALS
VOLLEYBALL

DAILY

1. Diaphragm Breathing - 10 times
2. Diaphragm Release - as needed
3. Sacral Rock
4. Respiratory Spinal Extension
5. Two-Minute Energy Balance
6. Warm-Up for 5 minutes (jumping jacks, jump rope) and stretch for 30 minutes
7. Visualize your event

PRE.COMPETITION

1. Pre-oxygenate - Diaphragmatically Breathe as much as possible
2. Acupressure Points - **PUMP FIRMLY**

Lg.I.4	T.W.4	C.V.17
Lg.I.10	St.36	K. 3

3. Neuro-Lymphatics - **RUB FIRMLY**

   Diaphragm

   Quadriceps
4. Neuro-Vasculars - **HOLD LIGHTLY**

   Knee - Hold hands lightly behind knees for 30 seconds to 1 minute. Infuses muscles with blood.

POST-EVENT

1. Warm-down and stretch for 30 minutes
2. Then do **COOL DOWN ACUPRESSURE POINTS**
3. Neuro-lymphatics - **RUB FIRMLY**

Quadriceps	Buttock muscles (Glutes)
Hamstrings	Low Back

4. That night take a **HOT EPSOM SALTS BATH** to relax the muscles
5. Drink plenty of water
6. Get plenty of rest
7. Get a massage

SAMPLE RITUALS
SKIIER

DAILY

1. Diaphragm Breathing - 10 times
2. Diaphragm Release-as needed
3. Sacral Rock
4. Respiratory Spinal Extension
5. Two-Minute Energy Balance
6. Warm-up 5 minutes (jumping jacks, jump rope, etc.) and stretch for 30 minutes prior to competition
7. Visualize the race

PRE-RACE

1. Pre-oxygenate your lungs -Diaphragmatically Breathe as much as possible.
2. Release Diaphragm - if needed
3. Acupressure Points - **PUMP FIRMLY**

   Lg. I. 4   T.W. 4   St. 36

   Lg. I. 10   C.V. 17

4. Neuro-Lymphatics - **RUB FIRMLY** after warm-up, 10-20 minutes prior to competition.

   Diaphragm   Hamstrings

   Quadriceps   Low Back

   Buttock muscles (Glutes)

5. Neuro-Vasculars - **HOLD LIGHTLY**

   Knee - Hold hands lightly behind knee for 20 seconds to 1 minute. Infuses muscles with blood.

6. Massage Warm-up

   Rub vigorously sides of Knees (medial and lateral collateral ligaments)) and above and below the Knee-cap (Quadricep tendon).

SAMPLE RITUALS

SKIIER

POST-RACE

1. Neuro-lymphatics - **RUB FIRMLY,** 1 - 5 minutes

   Quadriceps   Hamstrings

   Buttock muscles (Glutes)   Low Back

2. Acupressure, **COOL DOWN POINTS**

3. That night take a **HOT EPSOM SALTS BATH** to relax the muscles

4. Drink plenty of water

5. Get plenty of rest

6. Stretch for 30 minutes, holding each position for 1 minute

7. Get a massage

YOUR OWN PERSONAL RITUAL

Refer back to the different chapters and choose the techniques and points you need to **CREATE YOUR OWN RITUAL!**

DAILY

1.	Practice Diaphragmatic Breathing	(pg. 10)
2.	Diaphragm Release — as needed	(pg. 22)
3.	Sacral Rock	(pg. 30)
4.	Respiratory Spinal Extension	(pg. 32)
5.	Two-Minute Energy Balance	(pg. 35)

NEURO-LYMPHATIC POINTS (pg. 61)

1. _____
2. _____
3. _____
4. _____
5. _____

ACUPRESSURE POINTS (pg. 45)

1. _____
2. _____
3. _____
4. _____
5. _____

NOTES TO MYSELF

_____

_____

_____

_____

_____

_____

YOUR OWN PERSONAL RITUAL

Refer back to the different chapters and choose the techniques and points you need to **CREATE YOUR OWN RITUAL!**

DAILY

1.	Practice Diaphragmatic Breathing	(pg. 10)
2.	Diaphragm Release — as needed	(pg. 22)
3.	Sacral Rock	(pg. 30)
4.	Respiratory Spinal Extension	(pg. 32)
5.	Two-Minute Energy Balance	(pg. 35)

NEURO-LYMPHATIC POINTS   (pg. 61)

1. _____
2. _____
3. _____
4. _____
5. _____

ACUPRESSURE POINTS   (pg. 45)

1. _____
2. _____
3. _____
4. _____
5. _____

NOTES TO MYSELF

_____
_____
_____
_____
_____
_____
_____

APPENDIX III – TESTIMONIALS

PIKES PEAK ASCENT, AUGUST 20, 1988, 14,110 FEET - BESS JAMES

BESS JAMES, AGE 79, MASTERS RUNNER

Bess has been a client of mine for 4 years. She is one of a kind! Bess uses my techniques whenever she runs a marathon and she especially used it here, at Pikes Peak. Bess is the oldest women to finish the race in 25 years!

BESS'S RITUAL

PRE-RACE

1. Diaphragm Breathing - as much as possible to oxygenate her lungs
2. Neuro-Lymphatics

    Diaphragm   Quadriceps
3. Acupressure points

    Lg.I. 4   St. 36   T.W. 4

    Lg.I. 10   C.V.17

RUN

"I pumped on C.V. 17, Lg.I. 4, and T.W. 4 the whole way up. I was always doing something. Either rubbing up and down my sternum or along my lower rib cage."

"When I reached the top, my legs did not hurt at all! No soreness and I wasn't even tired! Whenever I started to get tired, I rubbed my points, and I was revived!"

RECOVERY

1. Drank lots of water
2. Rubbed the lymphatic point for the quadriceps
3. Lightly held the COOL DOWN ACUPRESSURE POINTS, Heart 7 and the Emotional Stress Points
4. Took a Hot Epsom Salts Bath and got a good nights sleep.

"The next morning, I felt like I didn't even do the race. Couldn't believe I felt so good. Felt great, Fantastic!"

Thank you Bess for trying my system.

Congratulations, Bess

Bess holds 2 World Records, 3000 meters and 5000 meters and 4 American Records, 1500, 3000, 5000, and 10,000 meters. She also holds the record for a 30k via the SCATAC Championships. She was also named 2nd place in RUNNING TIMES as RUNNER OF THE YEAR IN THE 75-79 age group in 1988.

TESTIMONIALS

"It is important for me to make sure to activate the diaphragm by breathing before proceeding through the rest of the ritual. When I don't breathe first, my sacrum doesn't fall into place, even with the rocking and the spinal extension.

"Lying down works best for me when I can. But when I am running, my stomach locks up (it feels like I am not getting any air), or I get a cramp. Standing, walking, or running slower and doing the Diaphragm Release will get rid of any cramp and open up my airway so I can breathe."

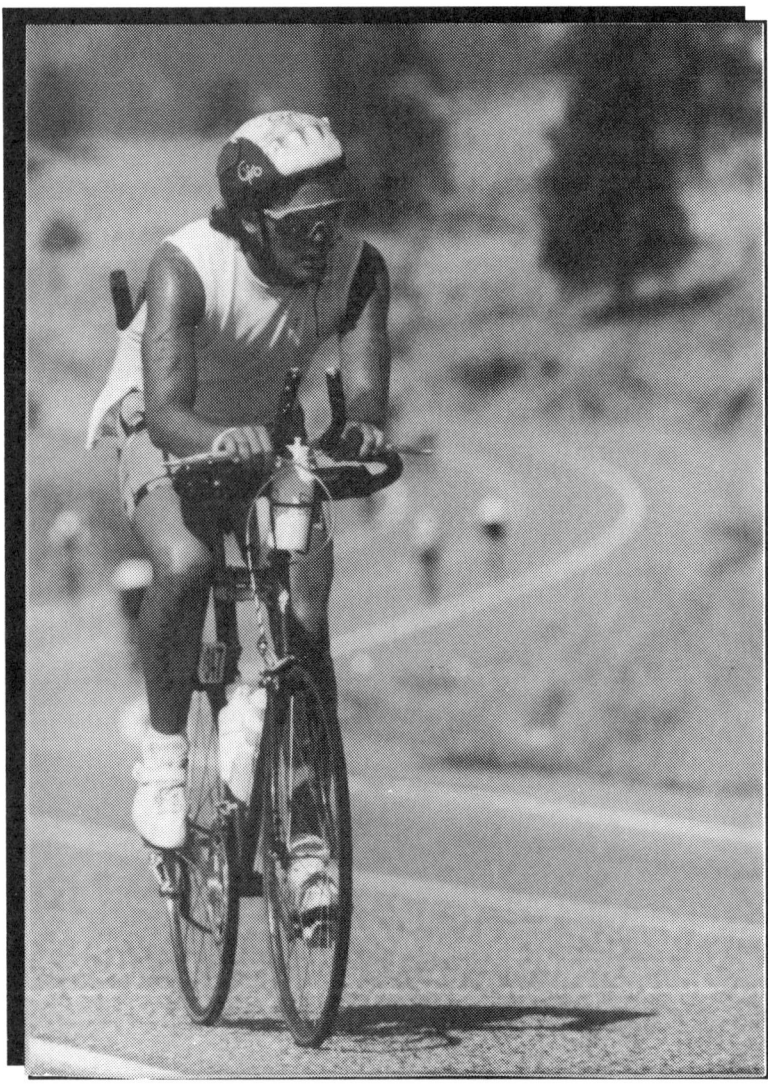

David Hemingway
27 years old
Canadian Ironman, 1988
Winner of 4 Triathlons
13th in World Triathlon
Championships - Nice
11th in National Ultra
Championships
2:40 Marathon
7:50 50 miler

TESTIMONIALS

CANADIAN IRONMAN, 1987 • David Hemingway

DAVID HEMINGWAY, AGE 25, ATHLETIC-TRAINER

David was the first athlete to test my system out in a major competition. Here are David's experiences and how it was able to help him in this race.

DIAPHRAGM RELEASE

"It's important for me to make sure and activate my diaphragm before preceding through the rest of the ritual. When I don't breathe first, my sacrum doesn't fall into place even with the rocking and the spinal extension.

"Lying down works best for me, but that's not always possible. When I'm running and my stomach locks up (it feels like I'm not getting any air) or I get a cramp, standing, walking or running slower and doing the Diaphragm Release gets rid of the cramp and opens up my airway."

SACRAL ROCK

"I need to make sure NOT to lean too far back, and to stay up high on the end of my tail bone. When rocking, I don't just twist my hips and keep my upper body still. It's important to rock both the upper and lower body as one unit."

SPINAL EXTENSION

"To get the most out of this technique, I need to make sure and exhale when pulling my knee over. Also, it is best to bring my knee up as high as possible to the opposite shoulder (left knee/right shoulder) -NOT just straight over to get my back to stretch more effectively."

ATHLETIC RITUAL IN TRAINING

"I went through the ritual before each workout while I prepared for my race. I never had any back soreness at all, where as before I experienced lower back pain after long bike rides and runs. Ten days before the race I spent much more time on each aspect of the ritual, focusing mentally on the function of each technique and visualizing what was happening to my body. I could definitely get greater benefits when I spent more time concentrating on what the technique was actually doing."

TESTIMONIALS

CANADIAN IRONMAN, 1987 • David Hemingway

SWIM

"The start of the swim was very smooth. But about 1500 meters into it, I started to get a cramp in my stomach. I tried to swim with it, but it really started bothering me. So I began breathing faster than normal - emphasizing belly-breathing and trying to open up my diaphragm. Cramps in your stomach while swimming are especially hard to get rid of because your body is extended. I didn't have any problem after 2000 meters as long as I overemphasized my breathing (especially exhaling) to keep my diaphragm open."

BIKE

"In the transition from swimming to biking, I did the Sacral rock and the Spinal Extension. Early on in the bike, I made sure to pump Lg. I. 4 and Lg. I. 10 to open me up until I was used to the change of pace. Also, I rubbed my neuro-lymphatics for the quadriceps located along my lower rib cage, to get rid of the poisons and toxins that make your legs feel heavy on the bike after swimming. All in all my bike ride went pretty well, as I used this ritual: Kidney 27, Lg. I. 4, Lg. I. 10, Central Vessel 17, and tapping my thymus. I did all these points at one time throughout the race. I couldn't feel the affect immediately, but after about 5-10 minutes, I felt like someone who had been hungry for a long time, run out of energy then finally got to eat something. The energy didn't come in a burst, but more slowly, in a way that enabled me to focus and relax and NOT feel uncomfortable."

RUN

"I did the Sacral Rock and the Spinal Extension after the bike to run transition. My back was hurting me at this point, but after doing the ritual, I felt as though I could breath again and my back was where it was supposed to be.

"The beginning of the run was okay but the drink mix they had at the aid stations was too concentrated and it really affected my stomach. It wanted to just close down. I felt like I couldn't breathe and I was on the verge of having cramps. I truly feel that if I hadn't done the Diaphragm release, I wouldn't have been able to run at all. Even though I was uncomfortable, I could still perform. I feel, especially in triathlons, that people have problems with their stomachs locking up on the "run" portion of the event. And if you don't breathe correctly, you'll get cramps from being bent over for hours on a bicycle. Through the run I rubbed neuro-lymphatics for the diaphragm and the quadriceps and pumped acupressure points Lg. I. 4, Lg. I. 10, C.V. 17, and T.W. 4."

TESTIMONIALS

CANADIAN IRONMAN, 1987 • David Hemingway

RECOVERY

"After the race I was very disappointed because I really felt I could finish in under or around 10 hours. But your rituals helped me pull myself out of some very tough spots (i.e.. cramps in the swim, losing energy very quickly in the last 20 miles of the bike ride, and stomach problems in the run). And most important, beyond the physical benefits, your rituals gave me the confidence that I could pull myself up and out when I was going under. This confidence grew as I saw immediate results from my breathing and from rubbing neuro-lymphatic points and acupressure points. Even though my final result was disappointing, I feel that your rituals were a major factor in getting me through the first 5/6 of the race as fast as I did.

"I wasn't able to go through a complete cool-down ritual because I was in the medical-tent and then had to catch a plane home with only five hours sleep. Needless to say, it was a long day! But I did manage to go through all of the Energy Balancing techniques even as I traveled. The week after the event I was never really sore in my muscles and joints. The only real-impact of the race was on my energy level — *for a few days*, I didn't feel like doing any heavy exercising.

"I truly believe in this whole concept of yours, Kate. I think it's marvelous that we are finally getting to the point of combining Eastern-spiritual awareness with the external power of our Western style sports activities."

Triathlon Credits:
Winner of 4 triathlons
l3th in World Triathlon
Championships - Nice 1986
llth in National Ultra Championships
2:40 Marathon
7:50 50 miler

IRONMAN

The world-class Ironman competition is held annually in Kona, Hawaii. It encompasses a 2.5 mile swim, 112 mile bike ride, and a marathon, 26.2 mile race. It is an incredible feat for any athlete who completes this demanding course. Oct 14, 1989, a full moon, weather conditions were perfect! The water was like glass and not a wisp of wind was blowing. The temperature was 80 degrees, with cloud cover making the scenario ideal for breaking records. However, my client just wanted to finish in style and recover quickly and without the usual after-effects of this challenging but grueling endeavor.

Is there a **"Secret Weapon"** which can accomplish that? The good news is *yes!*

I took my Athletic Rituals to Kona, to meet new athletes in which to try out my system. Scott Tinley (a fellow San Diegan) had agreed to try the Ritual at the Alcatraz Triathlon in San Francisco 2 weeks prior to the Ironman and was pleased with the results.

"This was the first time I wasn't winded coming out of the water!"

"My legs felt great and they never got heavy or tender."

Scott tried the Ritual for the second time in Kona. Like so many others he set a new personal record, but without paying the price of extreme tenderness in his legs. He rubbed his pressure points continuously every 1 — 2 miles to increase his stamina and endurance and to rid his body of waste build-up.

Scott, along with Joe Kilmer, John Carey, Bill Brown and Mike Baker, all used my system. From what they describe, their results were awesome!

In the following pages you can read how they used the Ritual to make it through this marathon event with ease and style. It worked for them, even better than I'd hoped, and if you try it, I know that you,too, will be amazed and delighted with the results.

TESTIMONIALS
SCOTT TINLEY

SCOTT TINLEY, AGE 32, PROFESSIONAL TRIATHLETE, TWO-TIME IRONMAN CHAMPION

SCOTT'S RITUAL

I met Scott four days prior to the Alcatraz Triathlon in San Francisco Sept., 1989, two weeks prior to the Ironman. Scott listened to me about my techniques and agreed to try them. Scott was able to master these techniques, as he practiced them everyday to make them second nature.

"I found these techniques to be simple and easy to learn. Not technical at all. There was no right way or wrong way to do them, which is why it is so easy."

DAILY

1. Diaphragmatically breathe — Practiced all the time
2. Sacral Rock
3. Respiratory Spinal Extension
4 Diaphragm Release — when needed
5. Two-Minute Energy Balance

PRE-RACE — SWIM

Diaphragmatically breathed — Pre-oxygenated his lungs as much as possible.

Pumped acupressure points Lg. I. 4 & 10, T. W. 4, St. 36, K. 3, and C.V. 17.

Rubbed neuro-lymphatic for the diaphragm.

"This was the first time I wasn't winded coming out of the water!"

TESTIMONIALS
SCOTT TINLEY

BIKE

Scott eliminated Steps 2 and 3 because of the speed factor.

RUN

Rubbed the neuro-lymphatics for the diaphragm and the quadriceps.

Pumped acupressure points Lg. I. 4, T.W. 4.

During the run, Scott noticed his legs didn't get that heavy feeling which usually slows him down.

"I felt very strong going into the race and Kate's techniques just helped me even more."

"My legs felt great and they never got heavy or tender."

TESTIMONIALS
SCOTT TINLEY

TWO WEEKS LATER

OCT. 14, 1989, IRONMAN

Scott used the Ritual outlined above in the Ironman. He consistently rubbed neuro-lymphatic points and acupressure points every 1 — 2 miles in the run.

Oct. 14th was a perfect day for breaking records and **Scott set a personal record of *8 hours, 35 min.; 59.9 seconds.* coming in 6th.**

Scott felt that one of the many contributing factors to his P.R. was the Ritual.

Later I gave Scott a massage. His legs were not as tender to the touch as he thought they would be.

Later that night Scott used my Herbal Healing Compress to soak his legs in — which helped to remove the soreness from his legs and speed, his recovery.

Thank you Scott, for trying my system.

Congratulations, Scott

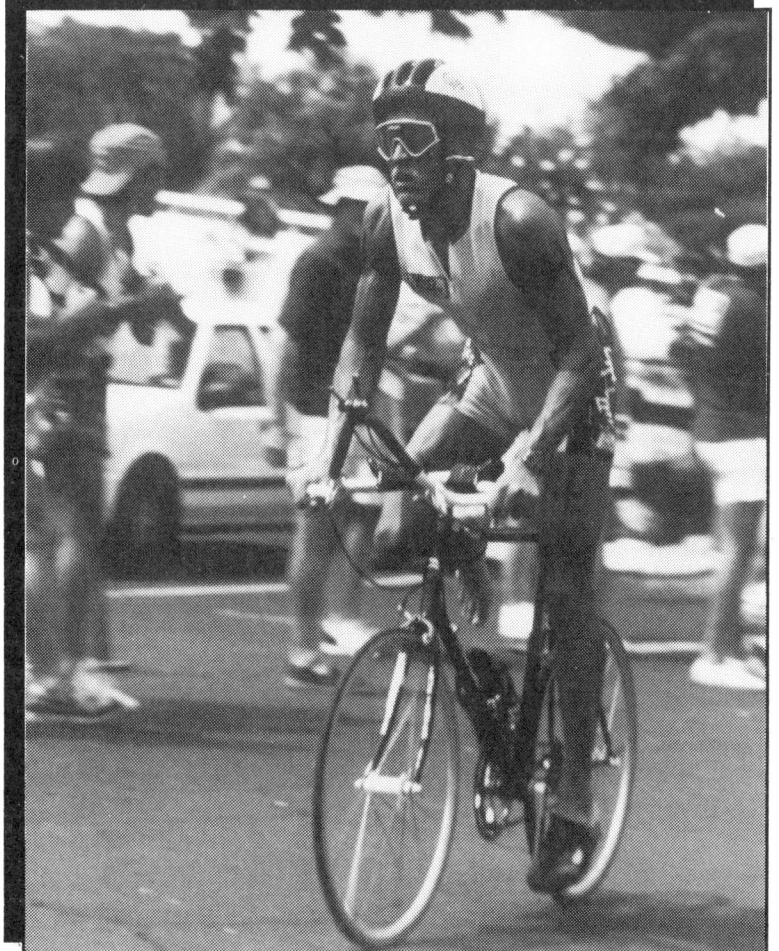

Photo by Russell Moore

TESTIMONIALS

IRONMAN, OCT. 14, 1989, KONA, HAWAII • Joe Kilmer

JOE KILMER, AGE 31, POLICEMAN

Joe received a Sports Massage from me 4 days prior to the Ironman. He had been experiencing a knee problem. This completely disappeared after a massage and the realignment of his sacrum.

PRE-RACE

"Awoke early on race morning.

"Diaphragmatic breathing - 10x's for 2 minutes.

"Sacral Rock - set sacrum.

"Respiratory Spinal Extension - stretch back muscles."

SWIM

"Prior to the start, pumped acupressure points Lg I. 4 and Lg. I. 10.

"Pre-oxygenated - Diaphragmatic breathing.

"Felt good after the swim."

SWIM TO BIKE TRANSITION

"While changing clothes, I practiced diaphragmatically breathing, rocked on my sacrum, and did the respiratory spinal extension and then started the bike ride."

ON THE RIDE

"During the 6 hour ride, in between eating and drinking, I was able to rub the neuro-lymphatics for the diaphragm, quadriceps and psoas.

"I still felt strong."

BIKE TO RUN TRANSITION

"Where the techniques really came into play was in the run portion. Repeated the same procedures as in the swim to bike transition."

TESTIMONIALS

IRONMAN, OCT. 14, 1989, KONA, HAWAII • Joe Kilmer

RUNNING

"While running, I was rubbing the neuro-lymphatics for the diaphragm, the quadriceps, and psoas. I pumped acupressure points Lg. I. 4, Lg. I. 10 and T. W. 4. All this was done constantly.

"Starting out on the run was tough at first and after that first hill I started rubbing my neuro-lymphatics for my quadriceps constantly.

"By mile 6 I was getting into it. I was doing about a 9 to 10 minute mile. I just wanted to finish so I was pacing myself.

"By mile 16, my legs were not sore, feeling heavy, or tired!

"By mile 18, I had plenty left and picked up the pace.

"In the past by mile 16, my legs were like lead and I was miserable.

"This time, it was just the opposite! These were my strongest miles!

"By mile 22, I felt so fresh, I picked up the pace again.

"The last mile and half, I felt fantastic!

"After the race, I felt so strong and knowing what I do now, using Kate's techniques, I feel I could have taken 40 to 60 minutes off my time.

"All I can say overall, is that I have run two previous marathons, and I was extremely sore for several days. I didn't even want to look at a pair of running shoes again!"

TESTIMONIALS

IRONMAN, OCT. 14, 1989, KONA, HAWAII • Joe Kilmer

RECOVERY

"That night after the massage Kate gave me, I felt good, tired but good.

"The next day, 5 minutes out of bed I felt fine. By the time the banquet arrived that night, I felt like I had not done it! I was thinking about next year and how I wish I could do it again!

"By Tuesday, 3 days after the race, I went running everyday, 5-7 miles and felt absolutely fantastic!

"Gauging by what I feel was an unbelievable recovery, I would recommend these techniques to anyone and have already done so. I still can't believe I feel this good, when I know friends of mine that are still not recovered a month later.

"These rituals are so easy to do. You don't have to think about it. There is no order, it is not technical, and it just becomes second nature. I didn't have to think about it, I just did it.

"Thanks Kate. You were a big part of probably the single greatest moment in my life. It was a great day for me. I've been wanting to do this race for so long. It was a dream come true for me and I feel I did it in style!

"You feel like you are running on all cylinders. I was very happy with my times. Had a great day!"

Joe finished the Ironman in 12 hours, 43 minutes and 48.9 seconds.

Congratulations, Joe.

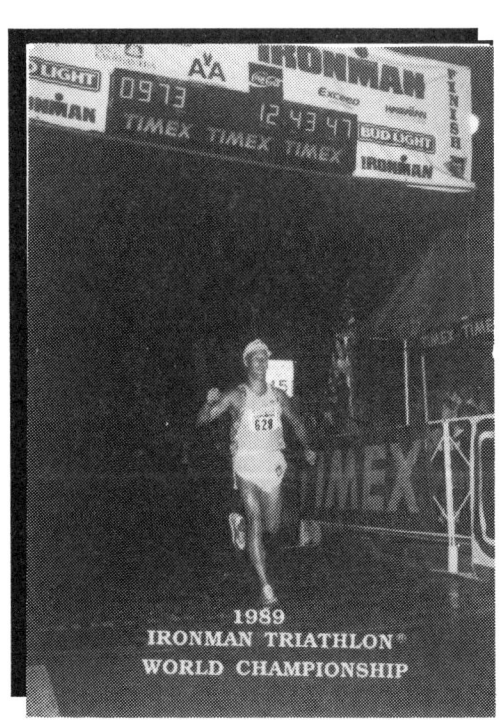

TESTIMONIALS

IRONMAN, OCT. 14, 1989, KONA, HAWAII • John Carey

JOHN CAREY, AGE 29, MECHANIC

JOHN'S RITUAL

PRE-RACE

John received a Sports Massage from me 4 days prior to the Ironman. He had been experiencing lower-back pain in training. I found his sacrum out of alignment and his low-back muscle in spasm. I was able to release the trigger points and spasm and stretch the sacrum back in place. I showed John how to work his low-back himself to keep it loose for race day.

"I was experiencing lower-back pain and you showed me where to apply pressure. I did this prior to race day and never experienced the back pain that was so difficult to deal with in training."

SWIM

Practiced diaphragmatic breathing to pre-oxygenate his lungs, Pumped acupressure points Lg. I. 4 and 10, T.W. 4. and St. 36. Rubbed the neuro-lymphatic for the diaphragm.

John had a right shoulder problem that was a recurrent problem for him.

"My right shoulder that had referred pain down my right arm never bothered me once in the swim, bike or run as it has in the past and is still fine to date!

"My swim time is usually about 1:10 to 1:20. To my surprise, I did it in 1 hour and felt great!"

TESTIMONIALS

IRONMAN, OCT. 14, 1989, KONA, HAWAII • *John Carey*

BIKE

John concentrated on his breathing all through the bike. He rubbed the neuro-lymphatic for the diaphragm which will keep this muscle from becoming tight and overworked. This will also keep this muscle relaxed so it doesn't tighten up on the esophagus and create a nauseous feeling.

"I frequently rubbed the upper center of my chest (neuro-lymphatic for the diaphragm which did seem to be the cause of relief to a very nauseous feeling. I did not want to drink or eat because of this feeling but dehydration was setting in. I began concentrating on rubbing my chest (sternum) and through this, I was able to eat and drink without nausea. I know this really did help, Kate because in training it would only get worse and I would end up having to lay down for an hour before the sick feeling would go away.

"I felt good after finishing the bike to make a believer out of me in the system!" I was ready to run — not fast, just smart. I felt together."

John's bike time was right on target.

RUN

John concentrated on his breathing, rubbing neuro-lymphatic points for the diaphragm, quadriceps, and psoas all through the run.

"I usually have that nauseated feeling but this time I experienced no nausea, chest pains, fatigue or weakness, heaviness in my legs.

"The final 2 miles I felt strong enough to run in at what I felt was like a 10k race pace.

"Overall, my swim time was 10-20 minutes faster than I anticipated, my bike was right on target thanks to this system, and the marathon just under 4 hours."

TESTIMONIALS

IRONMAN, OCT. 14, 1989, KONA, HAWAII • John Carey

RECOVERY

"I received a massage after the race. Other than being only slightly stiff the next day and a sore knee for the following 3 days, my recovery I thought was remarkable!

"I see the system not only as a training aid, but an injury and discomfort preventor that will enhance performance.

"I've experienced enough to want to understand more!

"Thank you Kate. You shared a very special time in my life and thank you for your help."

This was John's first Ironman distance and first marathon. He finished 413th overall and 17th out of 70 Canadians.

His time was 10 hours and 38 minutes.

Congratulations, John.

TESTIMONIALS

IRONMAN, OCT. 14, 1989, KONA, HAWAII • *Bill Brown*

BILL BROWN, AGE 57, RETIRED

BILL'S RITUAL

Bill received a sports massage from me 3 days prior to the Ironman. I noticed that Bill was already a diaphragmatic breather. I just encouraged him to continue it through the Ironman.

Bill wanted something that would help his legs most of all. I showed him the neuro-lymphatics for the quadriceps.

"I certainly used your method of massaging the neuro-lymphatics during the event. Whenever my quadriceps felt tired or like they were going to cramp, I would start to rub under my rib cage and was able to continue with a relieved feeling."

"I know there is no secret formula to pump life into a used up and very tired body, but your method definitely helped!"

RECOVERY

After the race, Bill went to the med tent to be checked out. Received 2 bags of glucose, then a massage.

"The next day I felt quite good and 2 days after the event I went for a swim and a 4 mile run. My legs felt great!"

Bill finished in 7th place in the 55-59 division.

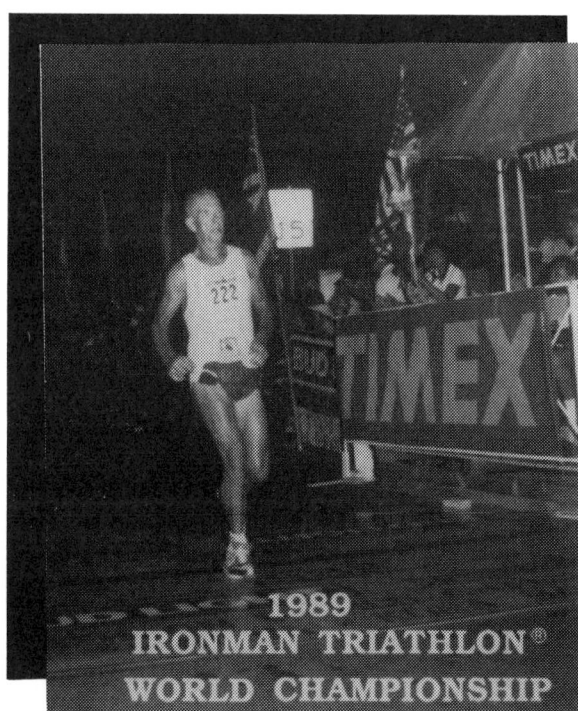

1989 IRONMAN TRIATHLON® WORLD CHAMPIONSHIP

Congratulations, Bill.

TESTIMONIALS

IRONMAN, OCT. 14, 1989, KONA, HAWAII • Mike Baker

MIKE BAKER, AGE 34, LAB. TECHNOLOGIST

This was Mike's second Ironman.

PRE-RACE

Mike received a massage 4 days prior to the Ironman. Mike had a sore hamstring and after the massage he had no further trouble.

PRE-SWIM

Practiced Diaphragmatic Breathing

Sacral Rock

Respiratory Spinal Extension

SWIM

Pre-oxygenated as he waited for the swim to begin

Pumped acupressure points - Lg. I. 4 & 10, C.V. 17.

Rubbed Neuro-Lymphatics for the Diaphragm and Quadriceps.

Finished in 58 minutes

BIKE

Rubbed the neuro-lymphatics for the Diaphragm and Quadriceps in-between eating and drinking water.

RUN

Rubbed the neuro-lymphatics for the Quadriceps and Diaphragm. Pumped acupressure points Lg.I. 4 & 10.

"Whenever I felt my legs getting heavy or sore, I would start rubbing the neuro-lymphatics for the quadriceps and soreness would just disappear. My legs would feel revived!"

"This year I was able to run the whole marathon - I felt a lot better and didn't feel spent."
I feel Kate's ritual contributed a lot to my outcome."

TESTIMONIALS

IRONMAN, OCT. 14, 1989, KONA, HAWAII • Mike Baker

RECOVERY

"Last year I was really sore and encouraged myself to take the elevator rather than the stairs. This year, the next day I felt great! A little sore but I got up and went out and "hammered" on the bike. I was never stiff or felt bad. My recovery was only ONE DAY and that was remarkable!"

Mike finished the Ironman in 10 hours and 50 Minutes.

Congratulations, Mike!

POST-SCRIPT

Mike returned home to El Paso, Texas and did 2 more events - Biathlons. A more intense competition and a higher level of intensity, he feels. He wanted to test the ritual in other races to evaluate its benefits. What he found was that it kept his legs fresh and revitalized. He rubbed the neuro-lymphatics to keep his legs from getting sore and acupressure points to keep his energy high.

"My recovery was truly remarkable thanks to Kate's rituals!"

"This is a great addition to my training, in competition and most important to my recovery!"

TESTIMONIALS
HERBAL HEALING COMPRESS

For athletes and week-end warriors or anyone who plays hard and even those who don't, John Finch turned me on to a herbal healing compress which is truly wonderful. I have used this mixture of herbs on myself as well as on many of my clients.

All I can say is that it's great! The next time you have an injury, try this "magic potion" in place of ice, or alternate it with ice, and see for yourself how quickly you regain strength, flexibility, and mobility!

TESTIMONIALS

"As a cyclist, I have found that using the Herbal Healing Compress that Kate recommended, along with her massage techniques, I've found I can significantly speed up my recovery time. An example of this was when I fell during a race. I skidded across the pavement on my hip. When I got home I found I did not have any broken skin, but I thought I would bruise badly and be very sore. I immediately made a tea of Healing Herbs and placed the compress on my hip. I did this 1-2 times a day for a week. I never bruised or was sore. My hip muscles never got tight. When I saw Kate the next week, I told her about the accident, but she couldn't find any evidence of the fall. That was remarkable!"

Steve Schraeder
Cyclist - Class 2

"I was involved in an automobile accident where I sustained a whiplash. Kate recommended the Healing Herbs for my neck. I used the healing herbs three times a day after receiving the whiplash. My shoulders and neck were very painful. It not only hurt, but it was painful to the touch. Healing herbs helped relieve some of the pain, also made the tissues not so raw, enabling my massage to be more effective."

Sara Berry
Nurse Staffing Coordinator
Whiplash Victim

TESTIMONIALS
HERBAL HEALING COMPRESS

"I was involved in an auto accident. After consulting with my Chiropractor, I was ok'd to see Kate. She recommended the Healing Herbs. I did so, anywhere from three to five times a day, within a two-week period. Kate was able to massage deeply into the muscle tissue by the sixth day. Kate said she had never seen anyone recover so quickly! I used these "herb packs" for four and a half weeks. The usage time varied depending on how I felt. Sometimes I felt more of a need. I was close to full recovery within 120 days. Many people suffer a long time with whiplash. I say "herb packs," massage therapy and chiropractic care helped me recover quickly!"

Melodie Tutt
Housewife
Whiplash Victim

"I myself was involved in a automobile accident while writing this book. I have used this compress numerous times and now I am using it on my neck. When I got home that night, I was starting to come out of the shock of the accident, and my neck and body were starting to hurt. I made up a tea of the compress and put it in my bath. I soaked in it for about 45 minutes, which relaxed me and calmed me down. Later I wrapped a compress around my neck to start a "flushing" of my tissues. I did alternate with ice at one point, which allowed my Chiropractor to work on my neck. I received immediate help from my Chiropractor and along with using the Healing Herbs, Two-Minute Energy Balancing technique, Acupuncture, and Massage, I was able to return to work within four days. My muscles never really got sore thanks to getting help as soon as possible. There is a lot of therapy involved in a whiplash accident, but the worse is suffering with the soreness in the muscles. I recommend all of these modes of therapy for the quickest possible recovery!"

Kate Montgomery
Sports Massage Therapist

APPENDIX IV — MASSAGE ORGANIZATIONS

The list below is just a few of the different massage organizations around the U.S.A. Please use them to find a qualifiied therapist in your area.

ALTERNATIVE HEALING HOTLINE
800/544-4980

AMERICAN ALLIANCE OF
MASSAGE PROFESSIONALS
3108 Route 10 West
Denville, NJ 07834
201/989-8939

AMERICAN MASSAGE THERAPY
ASSOCIATION
National Headquarters
Chicago, IL
312/761-AMTA

AMERICAN NUTRITIONAL
MEDICAL ASSOCIATION
Post Office Box 25113
Colorado Springs, CO 80936
719/591-2659

AMERICAN POLARITY THERAPY
ASSOCIATION
Post Office Box 44-154
West Somerville, MA 02144
617/776-6696

AMERICAN SHIATSU ASSOCIATION
Post Office Box 718
Jamaica Plain, MA 02130
617/236-5867

ASSOCIATED PROFESSIONAL
MASSAGE THERAPISTS AND
BODYWORKERS
1746 Cole Blvd., Suite 225
Golden, CO 80401-3210
303/674-8478

CALIFORNIA HEALTH
PRACTITIONERS ASSOCIATION
Post Office Box 90875
San Diego, CA 92109
619/459-7542

GREATER PHILEDELPHIA HOLISTIC
GUILD
13063 Townsend Road
Philedelphia, PA 19154
215/632-8244

HELLERWORK PRACTITIONERS
ASSOCIATION
Post Office Box 3228
Truckee, CA 95734
916/587-6715

INTERNATIONAL ASSOCIATION OF
INFANT MASSAGE INSTRUCTORS
Post Office Box 16103-D
Portland, OR 97216
503/253-9977

INTERNATIONAL MACROBIOTIC
SHIATSU SOCIETY
1122 M Street
Eureka, CA 95501-2442
707/445-2290

INTERNATIONAL MOVEMENT
THERAPY ASSOCIATION
Post Office Box 4777
Berkeley, CA 94704
415/525-6666

MASSAGE ORGANIZATIONS (cont.)

INTERNATIONAL MYOMASSETHICS
FEDERATION
5188 Picadilly Circle
Westminster, CA 92683
714/642-0735

INTERNATIONAL SHIATSU
ASSOCIATION
35 North Cass Avenue
Westmont, IL 60559
714/642-0735

JIN SHIN DO FOUNDATION
Post Office Box 1097
Felton, CA 95018
408/338-9454

MASSAGE THERAPIST ASSOCIATION
OF LOUISIANA
136 South Acadian Thruway
Baton Rouge, Louisiana 70806
504/387-0885

MINNESOTA THERAPEUTIC
MASSAGE NETWORK
Post Office Box 10767
Minneapolis, MN 55458
612/342-4341

MYOTHERAPY ASSOCIATION
OF TEXAS
403 Jordan Lane
Arlington, TX 76012
817/548-0104

NORTHWEST MASSAGE
PRACTITIONERS ASSOCIATION
1605 12th Avenue, Studio 30
Seattle, WA 98122
206/324-1491

ROSEN METHOD PROFESSIONAL
ASSOCIATION
2315 Prince St.
Berkeley, CA 94705
415/548-1205

SHIATSU PRACTITIONERS
ASSOCIATION
2309 Main St.
Santa Monica, CA 90405
213/396-4877

TENNESSEE ASSOCIATION OF
PROFESSIONALLY TRAINED
MASSAGE THERAPISTS
Post Office Box 16
Strawberry Plains, TN 37871
615/933-0521

UNITED STATES SPORTS
MASSAGE FEDERATION
120 East 18th St.
Costa Mesa, CA 92627
714/642-0735

THE AUTHOR
KATE MONTGOMERY

Kate Montgomery is a Holistic Health Practitioner whose specialties include Oriental Medicine, Therapeutic and Sports massage, and Applied Kinesiology, (Touch for Health).

She has a Holistic Health Practitioning degree from the Institute of Psychostructural Balancing — completing a 1000 hour program, with her internship focusing on Oriental Medicine. She is versed in deep tissue massage, sports massage, trigger point therapy and rehabilitative bodywork.

She is certified in Sports Massage through the Sports Massage Training Institute.

A NOTE FROM THE AUTHOR

I began my career in health care in 1971 as a respiratory therapist, and for the next twelve years I worked very hard to insure that my patients would make complete and lasting recoveries. But I often sensed that most of them didn't really understand how to take responsibility for their own well-being. Almost without exception, they would passively rely on medical personnel to "make them better." Although I was able to help these people in the short-term, I knew that as soon as they left the hospital (*or were back on their own*), they would slide back into their old bad habits and lose the progress they'd made.

In 1984, frustrated by my lack of ability to really make a lasting difference in my patient's lives, I entered massage school and there I discovered a whole new system of rules. It was there I studied the wholistic approach to taking charge of one's own life and health. As I began to learn more about my own body and how I could keep it healthy through preventive programs, I realized that here was a whole new world to explore.

I also realized that there must be others.like myself who were looking for alternatives to conventional medical care. So began my massage career. Because I am an athlete myself, I specialized in Sports Massage. Several of my colleagues formed the San Diego Sports Massage Team and we soon began volunteering our services at local 10k's, 1/2 marathons, marathons, triathlons, and swim meets, as we explored ways to speed recovery and improve performance.

In 1987, I started traveling to elite track and field events, from San Jose, Mobil Track and Field Championships, to Indianapolis for the Pan American Games.

At these events I was able to test some of the breathing techniques I had used as a respiratory therapist. The first thing I noticed, was that most of my athletes were NOT breathing properly and as a result, many of them experienced nausea and other symptoms after a race. I also discovered, by using applied kinesiology techniques, that many of them had muscles out-of-balance due to compensation, over-use and fatigue.

A NOTE FROM THE AUTHOR

In 1988, I began to put together a series of Rituals which I had found over the years to make a startling difference in my clients' performance. I went to Calgary for the winter Olympics and there I worked on Angela Schmidt-Foster, a Canadian World-class cross-country skier. She had been pushing herself to the limit and was seriously fatigued. I taught Angela how to breathe and balanced her muscles and within one hour she was already stronger and able to finish the finals the next day.

Two weeks prior to the summer Olympics in Seoul, Korea, I met Bob Ctvrtlik. He was a member of the USA Volleyball Team. Bob volunteered to try out my Rituals and I designed a Special Program for him. The results were fantastic!

In May of 1989, I traveled to Moscow with an international group of Sports Massage Therapists, to study the latest techniques and to create a network to further world peace. The methods I write about in this book are the result of all of these experiences, combined into a unique ritual. It has worked for clients, and I know, if you give it a chance, it will work for you too.

MY GIFT TO YOU

My last post-script is a simple prescription:

Be happy and smile a lot.

There's a poem I read everyday to help me keep going, and I'd like to share it with you. Whenever life is getting you down, remember:

"To solve each problem one at a time; to take each day as it comes.

*To stick to your goals, no matter what happens,
    and press on toward your dreams.*

*To keep your attention focused on the future,
    as you consider the solutions at hand.*

*To look for the bright side,
    even though it may be temporarily covered by a cloud.*

To smile often, even when a frown feels more natural.

To think of those you love, and know that they love you too...

*No matter how difficult it may seem,
    you have within you the power, the ability
    and the knowledge to make things better."*

By Lindsay Newman

GLOSSARY

APPLIED KINESIOLOGY	Study of movement of the muscles as applies to the evaluation of function.
ATROPHY	A wasting away due to non-use. Example: a wasting away of the muscles (shrinking) and bone that surrounds a joint due to injury or disease.
CO_2	Carbon dioxide - stimulates our respiration. An odorless gas. It is formed in the tissues and eliminated by the lungs as a waste by-product of respiration.
COCCYX	Four little bones fastened together below the sacrum that looks like a "tail," known as our "tailbone"
CONCEPTION VESSEL 2	On the midline of the abdomen, just above the pubic symphysis.
CONCEPTION VESSEL 24	In the depression above the chin, below the lower lip.
CROSS-CRAWL	An exercise to assist in the repatterning of certain central nervous system functions.
DIAPHRAGM MUSCLE	Muscle used in breathing. Separates abdominal cavity from the thoracic cavity.
FLIGHT/FIGHT SYNDROME	A syndrome synonymous with shallow breathing. Signs of anxiety, restlessness and tension caused by stress. Wanting to run away.

GLOSSARY

GOVERNING VESSEL 2	Top of the coccyx.
GOVERNING VESSEL 26	Below the nose, above the upper lip.
HEART	Pumps the blood through the body. Diaphragmatic Breathing helps to increase the oxygen supply to the tissues and venous return to the heart, allowing metabolism to work properly. It also encourages calcium and pH levels to remain normal.
HYPERVENTILATION	Shallow breathing.
KIDNEY 27	Located in the depression on the lower border of the sternum (breastbone).
KINESIOLOGY	Study of motion of the human body.
INNERVATION	The distribution or supply of nerves to a part.
LIVER	"Blood Reservoir." Moves several hundred milliliters of blood into the circulation of our tissues; cleansing system for the blood.
"LOCKED-IN" MUSCLE	When the muscle being tested has the slightest pressure applied to it and it feels strong and holds its position without waivering.
LYMPH	A transparent, slightly yellow liquid, derived from tissue fluids. It consists mostly of lymphocytes that help us fight infection in the body.

GLOSSARY

LYMPHATIC	Refers to lymph vessels.
MERIDIAN	A surface pathway that influences internal organs. The term comes from Chinese medicine.
MERIDIAN ENERGY	A vital force that flows through a pathway (meridian) that regulates internal function.
MIDLINE	An imaginary line that runs straight up the center of the body, front and back.
NEURO-LYMPHATIC REFLEX	Reflex points to stimulate lymphatic drainage in various areas throughout the body.
NEURO-VASCULAR REFLEX	Reflex points that influence circulatory function to parts of the body. Mostly found on the head, but are also located throughout the body.
OXYGEN	A gaseous element existing free in the air. It is an essential agent in the respiration of plants and animals.
PANCREAS	Regulates the enzymes for digestion of proteins, carbohydrates and fats.
pH	Partial pressure of hydrogen in the blood.
PLEXUS	A branch of a main nerve, subdivided into two or more nerves.
SACRAL PLEXUS	Located at the end of the spine in the sacrum; a network of nerves.

GLOSSARY

SMALL INTESTINE	Absorption of nutrients to the tissues of the body.
SOLAR PLEXUS	Located in the upper abdominal area; a network of nerves.
SPLEEN	"Blood Reservoir." Can increase in size and releases as much as 150 milliliters of blood to other areas of our body, especially during times of strenuous exercise. Acts as a cleansing system for the blood to rid it of toxins, bacteria and other harmful substances.
STOMACH	Stores food, mixes food with gastric juices, then slowly empties digested food into the small intestine.
"STRONG ARMING"	To hold a position while straining to do so.
STRONG MUSCLE	Has developed its full power; has an immediate locking when tested.
VENTILATION/PERFUSION RATIO	The ratio of air to blood mixture in our body.
WEAK MUSCLE	May or may not have developed its full power, but on manual testing, it does not neurologically function at its full capacity.

REFERENCES

Applied Kinesiology, Synopsis, *David S. Walther*, Systems D.C., Pueblo, Colorado, 1988.

Basic Human Physiology, *Arthur C. Guyton, M.D.*, W. B. Saunders Company, Philadelphia, Pennsylvania, 1971.

Breakthrough For Dyslexia and Learning Disabilities, *Carl Ferreri, D.C.*, Exposition Press of Florida, Florida, 1984.

Essentials of Chinese Acupuncture, lst edition, Foreign Language Press, Beijing, China, 1980.

Gray's Anatomy, *Henry Gray, F.R.S.*, Bounty Books, New York, New York, 1901.

Homeopathic Treatment of Sports Injuries, *Lyle W. Morgan, II, PhD*, Healing Arts Press, Rochester, VT, 1988.

HYPERTON-X, Total Body-Mind Integration, El Segundo, California, 1987.

Into Meditation Now, *Christopher Hills*, University of the Trees Press, Boulder Creek, California, 1979.

Medical Dictionary, Dorland's Illustrated, 25th edition, W. B. Sanders Company, Philadelphia, Pennsylvania, 1974.

Respiratory Physiology, The Essentials, *John B. West*, Williams and Wilkins Company, Philadelphia, Pennsylvania, 1979.

Science of Breath, *Swami Rama, Rudolph Ballentine, M.D., Alan Hymas, M.D.*, Himalayan International Institute of Yoga Science and Philosophy, 1981.

Stretching, *Bob Anderson*, Shelter Publications, Bolinas, California, 1980.

Touch for Health, *John F. Thie, D.C.*, De Vorss and Company, Marina del Rey, California, 1979.

YOUR OWN PERSONAL RITUAL

Refer back to the different chapters and choose the techniques and points you need to **CREATE YOUR OWN RITUAL!**

DAILY

1.	Practice Diaphragmatic Breathing	(pg. 10)
2.	Diaphragm Release — as needed	(pg. 22)
3.	Sacral Rock	(pg. 30)
4.	Respiratory Spinal Extension	(pg. 32)
5.	Two-Minute Energy Balance	(pg. 35)

NEURO-LYMPHATIC POINTS   (pg. 61)

1. _____
2. _____
3. _____
4. _____
5. _____

ACUPRESSURE POINTS   (pg. 45)

1. _____
2. _____
3. _____
4. _____
5. _____

NOTES TO MYSELF

_____
_____
_____
_____
_____
_____

YOUR OWN PERSONAL RITUAL

Refer back to the different chapters and choose the techniques and points you need to **CREATE YOUR OWN RITUAL!**

DAILY

1. Practice Diaphragmatic Breathing   (pg. 10)
2. Diaphragm Release — as needed   (pg. 22)
3. Sacral Rock   (pg. 30)
4. Respiratory Spinal Extension   (pg. 32)
5. Two-Minute Energy Balance   (pg. 35)

NEURO-LYMPHATIC POINTS   (pg. 61)

1. _____
2. _____
3. _____
4. _____
5. _____

ACUPRESSURE POINTS   (pg. 45)

1. _____
2. _____
3. _____
4. _____
5. _____

NOTES TO MYSELF

_____
_____
_____
_____
_____
_____